THE IN-BETWEEN

The
IN-BETWEEN

Unforgettable

Encounters

During

Life's Final

Moments

HADLEY VLAHOS, RN

BALLANTINE BOOKS

NEW YORK

Published in the United States by Ballantine Books,
an imprint of Random House, a division of
Penguin Random House LLC, New York.

BALLANTINE is a registered trademark
and the colophon is a trademark of
Penguin Random House LLC.

Hardback ISBN 978-0-593-49993-1
Ebook ISBN 978-0-593-49994-8

Printed in the United States of America on acid-free paper

randomhousebooks.com

6 8 9 7

FIRST EDITION

Book design by Barbara M. Bachman

To my husband.
I had been told my entire life that
my dreams were too big.
Then I met you, and you told me
to dream bigger.

Introduction

PEOPLE ARE OFTEN STARTLED WHEN THEY HEAR THAT I'm a hospice nurse. They ask me how I could do such difficult and sad work, day in and day out. While it's true that there are tough—and sometimes even devastating—moments in this line of work, there are many more beautiful ones. Moments of awe that make you stop and think about what it all means. Moments of deep love and the kind of wisdom that comes only from understanding that the end is near. So, while a lot of people might not understand why someone would choose to do my job, I consider myself lucky to be in hospice.

Hospice care occurs when people have been medically deemed to be near the end of life, and choose to stop treatment in a hospital or medical setting and, instead, spend those final days, weeks, or months in the comfort of their home, surrounded by loved ones. As a hospice nurse, I'm there to help guide both the patient and their loved ones through the process, and to keep the patient as comfortable and pain-free as possible. Hospice can last for up to six months, so in the process of this work, I get to know patients, their stories, their loved ones, and even their pets.

The stories in this book will share how inexplicable, powerful, and moving those moments leading from this life to whatever comes next (and I do believe there's *something* next) can be. I'm sharing these stories because there are so many misconceptions about both death and the process of dying. I get it. And I certainly don't have all of the answers, even though I've seen death enough times that I have a general idea of what to expect.

We don't tend to talk about hospice or death very much, but I know people are interested because I'm asked a lot of questions about it. Some people are generally curious about death and dying, while others have a specific reason to be interested in it, usually because they have a loved one in hospice, about to be in hospice, or who has been in hospice. Or maybe they're about to go into hospice themselves.

One of the questions I'm asked most frequently is how I became a hospice nurse in the first place. It's a natural question, especially for someone as young as I am—I turned thirty while I was writing this book, but I was twenty-four when I got started in the field, and way younger than everyone else I worked with. I still am. And my journey to becoming a hospice nurse certainly didn't follow a linear path. My childhood dream was to be a writer, and a nursing career never even crossed my mind when I started college. But looking back, I can trace how a series of events prepared me for this work.

For a lot of people, death can be a taboo or scary topic, but it wasn't in my family. My mom's parents were licensed embalmers and funeral directors, and my mom grew up at and around funeral homes and morgues. If you've seen the movie *My Girl*, then you understand what I'm talking about. It wasn't unusual for her to do her homework while bodies were being embalmed nearby.

Because of the family business, death was very literally a part of life, and so it wasn't unusual for dying and the topics surrounding it to become part of our dinnertime conversations. I grew up with the understanding that death was natural, and it felt normal to me, not scary or mysterious.

I was also raised with a fixed belief system about what happens *after* we die. I attended a private Episcopalian school in Baton Rouge, Louisiana, until I was ten, at which point my family moved to Destin, Florida, and we continued attending an Episcopalian church there. My class spent every Wednesday morning in the large cathedral on campus, and everything we learned was centered around the Bible. Even in music class, we only sang worship songs. My family life also centered around the church. We went every Sunday morning, and regularly attended social events there as well.

I believed every word of what I was told. I believed in Heaven, I believed in Hell, I believed in the Ten Commandments and everything else I was taught to believe. I didn't question, I just believed, and I didn't think twice about it.

Then, at fifteen, the world as I knew it ended.

It was a typical Friday night in high school, and just like most Friday nights, I was standing on the metal bleachers watching a football game. I had more than face paint on my freckled cheeks and held my best friend Hannah's hand, screaming along to the drum line as it played our school's fight song. I watched the football sail through the air, and then drop into my friend Taylor's hands, which caused us to cheer even louder.

And then, in a flash, two players from the opposing team hit Taylor, pushing him down onto the grass, and ending the play. I watched as Taylor struggled to get up, and then, once on his feet, appeared to shake it off and run over to the sidelines.

"I don't think he's okay," Hannah said, squeezing my hand harder.

"What? No, he's fine!" I protested.

A few moments later, an ambulance arrived at the sidelines and I watched in confusion as Taylor was taken away.

"Hadley, something's wrong," Hannah said again.

"I'm sure he just broke a bone or something. We can write something *super* funny on his cast."

Hannah nodded, and we turned our attention back to the football game.

Later that night, we went back to her house for a sleepover. We stayed up way too late giggling, painting our nails, and applying face masks. At one point, Hannah's mom stuck her head in the door and firmly told us, "Bed, *now*." Hannah rolled her eyes, but we obliged.

The next morning, we woke up and pulled on our Soffe shorts and T-shirts to head out to the school car wash, still groggy from staying up too late the night before. When we arrived at the parking lot outside the church, I realized everyone was crying. I stopped and looked at my friends, perplexed.

"He died," my friend Ashley said, looking up at Hannah and me through her tears.

"Who died?" I asked, still confused. I assumed it must be someone's grandparent.

"Taylor Haugen," she replied, choking out his name.

"He didn't die," I scoffed. "He's fine. I just saw him yester-day. I texted him."

I spun around and walked away from the group, already calling Taylor's number so I could prove to everyone that they were reacting to a stupid rumor. The phone rang and rang and rang, until it finally went to voicemail. I hung up and called Taylor's best friend, Chase, knowing he'd be able to clear things up. As soon as Chase answered, I said, "Everyone here is saying Taylor died. Please tell me what really happened. I know he didn't die."

Chase's voice sounded oddly flat. "He died. Last night."

I would later learn that Taylor's liver had burst when he was hit by the opposing team members. While he might have appeared to be okay as he got up and walked to the sidelines, the reality was that he wasn't okay at all. I didn't understand why Taylor couldn't be saved in the emergency surgery that was performed later that night. Isn't that exactly what the medical profession was supposed to do? *Save* people? Espe-cially young, strong, healthy people like Taylor.

For a long time, it didn't feel real. Sure, I knew this type of stuff happened, but it happened to *other* people, not to my friends. It felt like a bad dream, incomprehensible and shock-ing every time I realized anew that Taylor was gone—when he didn't walk me to fifth period, or show up for movie nights with our group of friends, or text me.*

---

* Taylor's parents established a nonprofit in his name, the Taylor Haugen Foundation, which started the #PledgetoProtect campaign and provides core guards for football players to prevent abdominal injuries. You can learn more at taylorhaugen.org.

Even after the initial shock had worn off, something in me changed after Taylor died. I had understood death, of course, but I understood death as something that happened at the end of life—not at the beginning. And not like this. For the next year, I was angry at everyone—at my friends who carried on with life like nothing had happened, at the football players who hit Taylor, and especially at the priest who preached about how loving God was. I knew that a lot of people turned to their faith in times of loss, but I just couldn't. I had too many questions. Gone was the unquestioning belief that had shaped my early childhood; my faith was severely shaken. Now I wanted answers, so I asked anyone and everyone who would listen how God could allow pedophiles and murderers to exist on this earth, but take my good-hearted friend before he could live out his dreams. People at church tried to pacify me by saying that Taylor was in a better place. I rolled my eyes in response, while my mom pinched my arm, hissing at me to "be polite."

The summer after I graduated from high school, I moved three hours away to Tallahassee to attend Florida State University. There, I joined a sorority, where I learned up close and personal how the college had earned its reputation as a top party school. I had continued going to church after Taylor's death despite the fact that I no longer wholeheartedly believed, but not once during college did I step foot inside a church. After having grown up in a strict and religious environment, I was suddenly free. Here there were no rules, and I could do whatever I wanted. I was drinking most nights and struggling to find meaning and purpose in life. Going from a highly structured schedule to having complete freedom and ownership of my own life proved to be challenging for me. I felt too guilty to call my family and admit what I was doing, so I pretended everything was great whenever we talked.

At FSU, I was seeing someone in the way you do as a freshman in college. We were young and reckless—and I got pregnant at nineteen, the summer before my sophomore year. In the instant I saw that positive pregnancy test, everything changed, and all of the plans I'd had for my life were suddenly upended.

My mom was supportive of my decision to have the baby but, beyond her and my friend Hannah, who had stayed in Destin to attend community college, I felt alone and afraid. While the rest of my friends returned to school for their sophomore year in college, I remained in my childhood home, trying to figure out how I was going to support myself and my child. My world got very small. Even now, at thirty years old, I still look young, so you can imagine the looks I got as a pregnant nineteen-year-old. It was easier to just not leave the house at all. People who had no vested interest in my situation had a lot of opinions, none of which were helpful or did anything in the way of alleviating my own fears and anxieties.

I WENT FROM BEING a normal college kid to a mother-to-be. I couldn't go back to FSU, and my plan to be a writer wasn't going to cut it to support both myself and a child. I needed to come up with a new plan—quickly.

And, with this, my life set off on a completely different

trajectory than I had intended. I did some research and learned that nursing, which required only two years of schooling and paid about $50,000 per year, was the best option for efficiently creating a scenario where I could support myself and my baby. Plus, the local community college offered a program. Pregnant and uncertain, I spent that summer and the next year taking the prerequisites to enter the nursing program, and the next fall I started my first semester of nursing school.

My son, Brody, was born on Christmas Eve in 2012. Those early years were a blur of hard work: trying to keep us afloat as I juggled raising my son, getting my nursing degree, and beginning a career. While those days were long and hard and intense, I proved to myself that I could do things I never would have believed myself capable of previously. I graduated on schedule in two years, with both a degree and a yearlong internship at a local hospital under my belt.

After graduation, I went on to work in immediate care for a few months, then a nursing home for almost a year. I would love to say that I was a wonderful, caring nurse right out of the gate but that's just not totally honest: I did my job and I went home. It wasn't until I worked hospice that my life truly began to change.

I made the jump to hospice six years ago and, looking back, I can see that I landed exactly where I was supposed to, doing exactly what I was supposed to do.

But, of course, there were a lot of twists and turns along the way, and a lot of stories that got me from where I began to where I am now.

I'm excited to share these stories with you. When I started working in hospice, I was still searching. I didn't know if I believed in a higher power, in something more. While I still don't have all of the answers, the one thing I can tell you for certain is that there are things that defy medical explanation, and that in between here and whatever comes next, there is something powerful and peaceful.

I've seen it with my own eyes, time and time again.

THE IN-BETWEEN

Glenda

M Y HAIR WAS STILL WET FROM THE SHOWER AS I stood in front of the television absentmindedly watching the news with my BEST NURSE EVER mug in hand. I was sipping my coffee when I felt a tug on my scrubs. Looking down, I saw Brody's big blue eyes peering up at me.

"Juice, please?" he said, shaking his empty sippy cup in his still-chubby three-year-old hands. I smiled and picked him up, placing him on my hip as I walked over to the kitchen. After giving him his juice, I tapped my phone to check the time. I needed to leave by 7:20 A.M. to make it to the office by 8:00. It was 6:40 now, which meant I had just enough time to finish getting both of us ready and fed.

My phone rang as I opened the refrigerator to grab some eggs. I looked down to see my manager Kristin's name flash across the screen. She never called this early. I wondered what was wrong.

"Hello," I answered nervously.

"Hey, you!" she greeted me, sounding like she'd had way

more coffee than me. "I need you to come with me to a patient's home. Check your email for the address. I'm about ten minutes away."

I quickly looked up the address, panicking when I realized that it was in a very nice part of town, just minutes from the beautiful white sandy beaches that Destin, Florida, is known for. Although I'd spent the latter part of my childhood in Destin, I now lived in the next town over, aptly named Niceville, in a little blue house that I had bought for Brody and me earlier that year. As a young single mom, I couldn't afford anything bigger or closer to the beach, but I was so proud of this home that I'd managed to buy for us a few months into my first nursing job.

"I'm at least thirty minutes away and need to drop off my son at daycare. Is that okay?" I asked cautiously, worried the delay would annoy her.

"No problem!" Kristin replied cheerfully before hanging up the phone.

Anxiety set in as I realized I needed to move quickly. I put the eggs back in the fridge, deciding to forgo breakfast altogether, twisted my wet hair into a low bun, and threw on my scrub top. After making sure Brody was dressed in the appropriate number of layers (because, yes, northern Florida *does* have a winter!), I stepped out into the crisp, cold air and headed to his daycare.

Brody's teacher barely looked up from her phone as I dropped him off at his classroom. "So sorry to bother you," I said, approaching her timidly, "but I didn't have a chance to feed Brody this morning. Can you make sure he gets breakfast?"

Without saying a word in response, the teacher rolled her eyes and let the kitchen know there would be one more kid than usual eating breakfast. I felt the familiar no-win pull between work life and mom life tug at my heart. One of the practical elements that appealed to me about hospice nursing is that it was generally an eight-to-five job, which meant predictability for my schedule with Brody, but not *every* day was like that, and apparently today was one of those days. It wasn't even 7:00 A.M. yet, and I already felt like a failure in the mom category, but I couldn't afford to lose my job. I was a few weeks into my new position as a hospice nurse, and in the process of training, which meant that I spent my days shadowing more senior nurses like Kristin as they visited patients. Keeping my manager happy had to come first.

I drove to the patient's home, passing many beautiful beach houses just like the one I had grown up in. I turned left onto Coral Cove, and saw Kristin's Hyundai sedan in the driveway of a beach bungalow with green shutters, surrounded by a few palm trees artfully placed around the front yard. The home wasn't imposing in the way I had feared. On the porch, two rocking chairs swayed back and forth in the breeze, and the lights that glowed from inside the house were warm and inviting. I took a deep breath.

Kristin met me in front of the house, her impeccably curled blond hair framing her face, which was beautifully made-up even at this hour. "Ready, Freddy?" she asked, flashing her perfect smile. I smiled slightly in return and nodded, feeling insecure in my wet bun and bare face.

The truth was, I didn't feel ready. As a hospice nurse, of course I knew that attending a patient's death was inevitable, but I hadn't had to face it yet. I had a sense this patient was going to be different.

As we walked up the concrete steps, a frazzled red-haired woman in her forties opened the door before we could even knock. She looked like she had just rolled out of bed, yet hadn't slept for a moment.

"Come in, come in," she said, waving us inside. I could smell coffee brewing in the kitchen as a barking teacup poodle ran up to us, pausing to sniff my brand-new sneakers, a gift from my mom to celebrate my new job.

"So, she's been talking to deceased loved ones?" Kristin asked the patient's daughter, Maria, who was now trying to herd the dog into a laundry room off the kitchen. Hearing this, I raised my eyebrows, my suspicions confirmed. This was not another "normal" visit, after all. Despite what movies and television might lead you to believe, most of a hospice nurse's day is spent driving from one patient's home to the next, where we spend thirty minutes to an hour checking in on the patient and helping their caregiver or family member with whatever they might need to keep the patient comfortable. Maria *did* need help, it seemed, but not in the usual ways of checking to ensure her mom had the proper medications, that her symptoms were under control, or routine wound care.

"If you want to call it that," Maria replied as she grabbed a coffee mug from the kitchen cabinet. "I call it being out of her damn mind. She's mostly talking to her sister, who passed before I was even born. Please make this craziness stop. I can't sleep." Maria took a long gulp of coffee, as if to emphasize the point. As she drank, I took a deep whiff, allowing the strong smell to help ground me as my mind buzzed with confusion.

"All she does is talk to herself nonstop. Y'all must have some medications to make her sleep. If not, I'm going to call 911."

"Okay, Hadley and I will go take a look at her," Kristin told Maria reassuringly.

As we walked down the hall, I began hearing the faint voice of a woman. We entered the bedroom and I took in the sliding glass doors that led out to a patio, a heavy wooden dresser and matching nightstands, and a smaller table next to the dresser, piled high with books. A large chandelier hung over it, beautiful and ornate. As my eyes scanned the room, they finally came to rest on Ms. Glenda, whose white curls were cut short to frame her face. She roared with laughter even though there was no other sound—or person—in the room.

I watched Ms. Glenda incredulously as she continued pointing and laughing at the air in front of her, seemingly unaware that Kristin and I were there.

"No, no, no!" she exclaimed. "I didn't say that. You are too much!" Her laughter echoed throughout the room.

Kristin walked up to her bedside and lightly touched her arm. "Hey, Ms. Glenda! It's Kristin and one of our newer nurses, Hadley." I stepped up to her bedside and waved awkwardly.

"Well, hey!" Ms. Glenda greeted us. "You'll have to excuse me, we haven't spoken in years."

"Who haven't you spoken to?" Kristin asked.

"Oh! I couldn't be any ruder, could I?" Ms. Glenda said with a heavy Southern drawl. "This is my sister. Do you need to take my blood pressure now, sweet pea?"

Kristin nodded and pulled out the blood pressure cuff

from her nursing bag. I stood nearby, looking on in confusion, stunned that she was so unbothered by the fact that we had just been "introduced" to an invisible, deceased sister. Before coming on as a hospice nurse, I had worked in a hospital, where Ms. Glenda would have been medicated with anti-psychotics before she could even finish her sentence.

After Kristin finished taking Ms. Glenda's vital signs and declared her numbers to be perfect, she went to grab Maria. For a moment, it was just me and Ms. Glenda. I wasn't sure what to do or say, so I met her eyes, half smiled, and awkwardly played with the zipper on my own nursing bag. Thankfully, Kristin was only gone for a moment, and once she returned to the room with Maria, she started laying out the "game plan."

"I know you're tired and concerned about your mom," she said to Maria. Then, turning to Ms. Glenda, she said, "And, Ms. Glenda, I know you have people you need to catch up with, so what we're going to do—as long as you two are okay with it—is initiate something called continuous care."

It's only at the point when the family caregiver can't handle a situation anymore that we initiate continuous care, where a nurse remains at the home round-the-clock either until the patient's symptoms are more manageable or the nurse is otherwise no longer needed. I hadn't been in a continuous care situation yet, and I was eager to see it performed and to learn all about the antipsychotic medications hospice used.

As Maria nodded in agreement, Kristin continued, "Hadley will be staying around the clock with you, at least until her shift ends, then another nurse will take over, and we will continue that cycle until things are more manageable for everyone."

Shocked, I gave Kristin a wide-eyed look and subtly shook my head to indicate that I wasn't ready to handle adjusting heavy medications on my own. She smiled back at me, reassuringly, and mouthed, "We'll talk." I tried to return her smile, but I was freaking out. I wasn't ready for this! Why had I thought hospice was the right fit for me?

As Kristin walked back into the hallway and motioned for me to follow her, I tried to act as calm as possible. I explained to her that I didn't have any experience with psychiatric medications for hospice patients.

I could tell Kristin was trying to hide a smile as she said, "No worries! You won't need to give any medications unless something changes. In that case, call me or the doctor."

Confused, I asked what she meant. How could we not give Ms. Glenda medication? Clearly, she was hallucinating heavily.

"She isn't hallucinating," Kristin explained. "She is crossing over and seeing her deceased sister. All you need to do is be by her side and ensure her safety so her daughter can rest."

I nodded my head like I understood, but I absolutely did not.

I had seen death when I was interning in the ER during my nursing school days a couple of years before, but that was nothing like this. Even though I understood what hospice was, it felt foreign not to be doing something to alleviate symptoms, and to be in an environment this quiet and calm. In hospital situations like the ones I'd been in up to this point, death was usually a quick, traumatic occurrence. There's a lot of chaos and frenzy, with up to fifteen people in a single room, running around, doing CPR, pushing medications, ventilating, and monitoring the patient for return of a pulse. The family is not in the room—or, if they are, they're quickly ushered out—until the patient dies, at which point they're called back in to say their goodbyes. When all is said and done, the nurses return to their station and move on to the next patient.

It's not that I wasn't affected by those deaths—I was. But the nurses I admired the most from my time in the ER could go from one death to the next like it was no big deal at all. Most doctors and nurses admired those who could do so. I wanted to be more like those nurses and be admired as well, but it was difficult for me to disconnect from the person in front of me.

This felt different—much more personal and intimate. After all, I was in Ms. Glenda's home, and her daughter was right down the hall, where she'd finally fallen asleep on the couch. It was quiet here, peaceful almost, with no chaos to be distracted by, and no specific timeline to anticipate.

A few minutes later, Kristin was gone and I was just . . . here.

I returned to Ms. Glenda's bedroom and grabbed one of the vintage chairs by the table, then asked if I could sit next to her. Ms. Glenda nodded yes without taking her eyes off the ceiling. After a few minutes of silence, I began reading my company's employee handbook on my tablet, unsure what else to do.

Twenty minutes or so later, Ms. Glenda turned her attention to me. "You think I'm crazy, huh?" she asked, smiling. She seemed to be almost entertained by the idea that I might think that.

Startled, I replied, "No, not at all!"

"It's okay, you know," she continued. "My daughter thinks I'm crazy."

I didn't respond because I didn't know how to. Ms. Glenda paused and readjusted herself in her bed before continuing, "I'm not crazy. My sister is standing right next to you."

Instinctively, I turned in the direction Ms. Glenda was indicating, but I only saw the bedside table. I nodded my head in response.

AS MS. GLENDA FELL asleep and the whole house quieted, I realized that my education hadn't prepared me for this. In the entire two years of nursing school, a total of one day had been dedicated to either home health or hospice, which are two totally different specialties—and I did home health. While home health patients are in their homes at the time of treatment, they're not dying, which obviously represents a significant difference between them and hospice patients.

I only really began to understand what hospice care was during my previous job, as a manager at a nursing home. The nursing home offered a program called respite, where we took in hospice patients for five-day periods when their caregivers needed a break. Aside from doling out medications, I didn't take care of the hospice patients even then, but I *did* see the hospice nurses who came in to care for the respite patients. I loved those nurses, and it seemed to me that they were able to focus on their patients in a way that I wasn't able to, which really appealed to me. While hospice nurses do have a case-load of approximately twelve to eighteen patients at any given time, they get to sit down and spend time with them—that's part of the job. In the nursing home, we had forty patients for every nurse, and I sometimes joked that I felt like a Pez dispenser running from one room to the next, because all this really left time for was doling out medications as necessary. As I ran down the hallways on my constant quest to give out medicine, I sometimes noticed hospice nurses sitting by their patients' bedsides, having a chat with them—it struck me as calm and peaceful, and I thought how nice it must be to get to connect with patients like that.

Every now and then, one of the hospice nurses would walk up to me, explain a situation with their patient, and then share their plan. Every time I asked a hospice nurse if I should call a doctor in response, they shook their head no, usually reply-ing that the doctor had already been alerted and things were under control. This, too, was so different from other types of nursing, where all hands are on deck trying to save a patient. Instead of trying to cure them with any and all treatments and medicines, hospice nurses were asking patients how they could make their quality of life better in the time they had left. I watched as patients spent time with their family instead of being shuffled from one appointment to the next. I saw how the hospice nurses went to great effort to alleviate their pain, but stopped there. This was how I felt medicine should be practiced.

The more I saw these hospice nurses, the more appealing their job looked. I decided to keep an eye out for openings

and even applied to some of the few-and-far-between oppor-
tunities that came up, but was unsuccessful. There were only
three hospice companies in my area at the time, each with
only three nurses on staff. Not to mention the fact that the job
listings that *did* come up required previous hospice experience, which was a bit of a catch-22. It was only through a
fortuitous (for me, at least) series of events that I finally landed
this one.

As I was working in the nursing home one day, there was
a soft knock at my door.

I called out, "Come in!" only to be greeted by a concerned-
looking woman. She explained that she was the daughter of
Tim, a patient in room 404 who had brain cancer and was
deteriorating rapidly. Hospice was supposed to arrive to admit
him an hour ago, but hadn't yet shown up or otherwise contacted them. I smiled as I told her that I would give the company a call, trying to disguise the anger that I could feel
heating up my body. It was clear that this woman felt vulnerable and didn't want to complain, but what a horrible situation she'd been put in. I'd seen patients have nothing but
stellar experiences with this company so far, but this wasn't
okay.

As soon as the woman left, I picked up the phone and
called the hospice company. The phone rang a few times before a woman who identified herself as Kristin answered. I
explained the situation and that I was feeling really upset for
Tim and his family. It just so happened that I'd had too much
coffee that day and not enough sleep the night before, so I
spoke more bluntly than I usually did. "Being admitted into
hospice has to be one of the worst feelings—and then feeling

like you don't even matter to the company on top of that has to make it worse. I'm sure there's a fine excuse, but it's still not okay that Tim has been treated this way."

Kristin explained that a nurse had left the company with no notice the weekend before, and as a result they had been unusually disorganized. "I can personally come admit Tim, though," she continued.

I exhaled in relief. "Sorry for giving you a hard time," I told Kristin as she hung up.

An hour later, Tim was admitted into hospice. The family looked happy as they hugged Kristin—who had come as promised—goodbye. As I watched her sanitize her hands from a few feet down the hallway, she caught my eye and walked toward me.

"Are you Hadley?" she asked.

"Yes. Sorry again about that."

"It's okay, truly," Kristin said. "I love how much you care about your patients." She paused for a couple of seconds before continuing. "Correct me if I'm wrong, but have I seen your name come through on an application in the past?"

I looked around, making sure that none of my co-workers were within earshot. "Yes, about six months ago. But I didn't get it."

"Are you still interested?" Kristin asked.

"Absolutely," I replied, trying to keep my voice from becoming high-pitched, like it tends to do when I'm excited.

"Can you come by after work for an interview?"

"I'll see you at five," I told her.

———

I HAD BEEN SO happy to get this job—I *was* so happy to have this job. And yet, as I sat here in this room with Ms. Glenda, I felt out of my depth. I wondered if I was right for hospice, after all. As I pondered all of this, I heard a stirring and looked down to see Ms. Glenda had opened her eyes and was looking up at me. "Hey," I said to her with a smile.

"I just had the loveliest dream," she sighed happily. "I was flying through fields of flowers with my parents. My mom looked so great. So young. I felt so much happiness and peace."

"That sounds amazing," I told her. It did.

Ms. Glenda exhaled and looked toward the wooden table by my side. "I see my sister is still here. She said she will be here with me until it's time to leave."

I looked at the wooden table, but all I saw was books. Intrigued, I asked Ms. Glenda where she was going.

"I don't know," she replied as she picked up the blanket covering her, and then placed it back down again. A few moments later, Maria came in. She walked over to the bed and kissed her mom's head, sighing as she told us that she felt much better after having gotten some sleep.

"Me too." Ms. Glenda smiled.

"Are you still seeing your sister?" Maria asked.

I braced myself for Ms. Glenda's response, knowing her daughter wouldn't like the answer.

"Nope. I guess I was just tired," she replied, turning her head to look at me. Her eyes bored into mine, daring me to correct her. I didn't say a word.

Maria exhaled and visibly relaxed as she held her mom's hand. She turned to me and thanked me for "fixing" her mom. I was unsure how to respond, so I said nothing.

While pretending to chart on my tablet, I continued to observe Ms. Glenda. I noticed that she kept glancing at the table by my side, and then up to the ceiling where the chandelier hung—the same spot she had looked at when she told me her deceased sister was still here. I kept looking over at that corner of the room, but I never saw anything. I wondered what she saw.

At noon Ms. Glenda's daughter said it was okay for me to leave. Back in my car, I called Kristin.

"Hey, Ms. Glenda and her daughter say they're okay now. I'm not sure what to do."

"Great! Did she need anything?"

"Nope, she just slept and then when she woke up, she told me she was still seeing her deceased sister, but then she lied to her daughter about it."

"She seems very aware of her surroundings and even aware of her daughter's feelings, in my opinion. Crazy how our loved ones come to get us, huh?"

"Is this normal?" I asked incredulously.

"Oh yeah, it happens all the time," Kristin answered casually. "So, in this case, don't actually choose the continuous care option since we didn't need to intervene. Our guidelines say that the nurses need to be providing symptoms management at least once per hour in order to call it continuous care. This was a best-case scenario where we didn't need to do that, so we'll just call it a longer nurse visit instead."

After agreeing and hanging up the phone, I stared at the driveway in front of me, feeling dazed. There's no way Ms. Glenda was *actually* seeing her deceased sister, right? I pulled out my tablet again, scrolling to her chart to look at the most recent doctor's note: *This is an eighty-six-year-old female with metastatic melanoma who adamantly refuses further treatment after surgery was recommended. After extensive discussion with the patient, who is alert and oriented, we have decided to refer to hospice services.*

Skin cancer is not something that causes confusion or hallucinations. I scrolled over to the latest CT scan, looking for another explanation. I found a scan from just a week before and began reading: *Large mass of porta hepatis nodes associated with marked irregular mural thickening of small bowel in the LIF with resultant luminal dilatation. No features of intussusception.*

Basically, the cancer had spread to her gastrointestinal area—but that still didn't explain the confusion. I stared out the window, baffled. It made no sense.

I figured there had to be some explanation for this that I hadn't yet learned. Hospice training consists of a week on the computer followed by direct training with a nurse, during which nurses new to the field are given a computer course and a book to read. Most of that training involves charting, which is an important part of hospice nursing and complying with Medicare guidelines. (And it's deeply complex—I would say it took me about three years before I felt like I really had a grasp on these guidelines.) After that, everything else is learned through shadowing, just like I'd been doing with Kristin that day. It might sound like a surprisingly little amount of training but, in my opinion, it's adequate. There are so many different scenarios to experience as a hospice nurse, and a book or course is never going to be able to teach them all. That knowledge has to be gained firsthand, through shadowing, and then over time doing the actual work.

I was scheduled to spend the rest of the afternoon shadowing a nurse named Amanda, so I put down my tablet with a sigh and drove to meet her at her patient's home. After watching Amanda complete a regular visit, I asked if she had seen Ms. Glenda before.

"Yes, I admitted her. Isn't she so sweet?"

"Super sweet," I agreed. "But she says that she saw her deceased sister. Did she seem confused to you?"

"Oh, no, she could answer all my questions when I asked if she knew where she was, who the president was, and what her name was. I was impressed by the president one, because she could even tell me that it was currently Obama but it was about to change—so no, she definitely wasn't confused."

"Huh," I said, incredulous. "So, some people really do see deceased loved ones? This is a normal thing?"

"Yup," she replied, "they all see the same thing. It doesn't matter their race, religion, or any other factor you could think of."

I nodded and tried to appear nonplussed, but my mind was racing. Why were all the nurses acting so casual about this?

That afternoon, Amanda and I called the night-shift nurse to give her a report on the day's patients, and she, too, was unfazed by Ms. Glenda's behavior.

"So, don't be surprised if you need to go see her tonight," Amanda told the nurse. "If she doesn't call, Hadley will go see her first thing tomorrow morning."

———

SHE DIDN'T CALL, so the next morning I arrived at Ms. Glenda's house promptly at eight.

Ms. Glenda was still asleep as I entered her bedroom and quietly placed my nursing bag on the floor. "Hey, Ms. Glenda, it's Hadley," I greeted her, peeling back her covers to reveal her arms. They were even paler than yesterday and tinted blue now. I touched her right arm, which was ice-cold. Gently, I said again, "Ms. Glenda?" I pulled out the stethoscope that I had stuffed into my scrub pocket and held it to her chest. Her heart was beating slowly, and so faintly that it was hard to hear. I placed my automatic blood pressure cuff around her arm and pressed the start button. It beeped and began inflating, the loud motor the only sound in the room other than Ms. Glenda's shallow breathing. I watched as the cuff deflated and attempted to inflate again, only to stop a few seconds later before it flashed ERROR twice and then turned off.

"Ms. Glenda, I'm going to check that bandage on your back," I said loudly this time. I turned her tiny frame over. The outline of her pillow had made an indentation on her upper back, but her dressing was clean. It's common for older people to get skin tears and bedsores, which can quickly become infected if they're not treated, so we're constantly on the lookout. I moved the pillow and placed it under her rib cage, then slowly lowered her body back down to the bed, positioning her so that she was slightly on her left side.

Through all of this, Ms. Glenda didn't move or make a sound. She was likely in a coma. I stepped into the hallway where Maria was standing and broke the news as gently as I could. Tears instantly spilled down her cheeks.

"What do I do?" she asked.

"I think you should talk to her, tell her how much you love her. I learned in school that people can still hear you, even if they can't respond."

Maria nodded and wiped her face with the back of her hand. I watched as she knelt at her mom's bedside and began to lovingly stroke her white curls away from her face.

"Momma, it's me. I'm sorry I was so harsh yesterday. I just feel so lost. You taught me everything I know except one very important thing: You never taught me how to handle losing the most important person in my life. What am I going to do without you?"

I felt tears forming as I watched the two of them. And then Ms. Glenda took in one breath, much louder than the others before it. Was this her last breath? After what seemed like a lifetime but was probably only a minute, Ms. Glenda took another loud breath, followed by a long pause.

Her daughter laid her head on her mom's arm. "You can go be with your sister," she sobbed. "I know you miss her. I miss you already, Momma. I love you."

Ms. Glenda took a smaller, calmer breath, and then everything went quiet. After a few moments, her daughter realized it was over. She searched her mom's face, looking lost. Instinctively, I reached over and placed my hand on Maria's shoulder. She responded by placing her hand on mine. We stayed like that for a moment; I didn't want to be the first one to move. After a few minutes, Maria turned to me.

"Now what?"

I wasn't sure. This was my first time handling a death alone and I suddenly couldn't remember any of my training.

"Let me check really quickly. Sorry," I muttered as I moved toward my bag. I rifled through my papers and found the checklist labeled "Steps for Patient Death." I quickly flipped to Step One: *Listen to the patient's heart for two minutes. If there is no heartbeat then look at the time and call time of death.*

I turned to Maria. "I have to call time of death now. I don't think I have to say it out loud, but are you okay being in here while I do that?"

"Yes," she replied. "But say it out loud. I think it will help it feel real to me."

"Okay," I said, putting my stethoscope into my ears. I walked over and held it firmly to Ms. Glenda's chest. Complete silence. I looked at my watch and waited for the second hand to make one full loop. Maria stood at my side. The light from the chandelier flickered off and I glanced up at it instinctively, missing the moment when the second hand hit the twelve, marking the first minute. Maria frowned in confusion. I didn't say anything as I continued listening for a heartbeat, determined not to miss the mark this time. As I watched the second hand, the chandelier flickered once again, then came back on. Two full minutes had passed without my hearing a heartbeat.

I looked at Maria and she gave me a reassuring nod as if to say, *I can handle it.*

"Time of death: 8:42 A.M.," I whispered.

Just then, there was a loud pop in the corner of the room. The chandelier had burned out, leaving us in complete darkness.

Carl

A FTER ABOUT EIGHT MONTHS OF SHADOWING AND being shadowed, I was ready to take on my first patient solo. I was both excited and nervous as I knocked on Mr. Carl's door. Although I'd practiced all of the essential skills of hospice nursing, I knew there was only so much I could prepare for. At some point sooner or later, I would find myself in a situation I had no previous experience with.

As we stood on Mr. Carl's doorstep, Travis—a hospice nurse who was moving up to a manager role and transitioning some of his patients over to me—gave me the rundown. He had been caring for Mr. Carl, who had congestive heart failure, for four months. Travis told me that Mr. Carl's wife was a nurse who liked to weigh in on medical decisions. I nodded but felt my heart rate speed up.

Veteran nurses tend to "eat their young," often bullying the less experienced nurses. I learned about this phenomenon early on in nursing school. Some veteran nurses rolled their eyes when interns like me were assigned to shadow them. Others showed even more obvious signs of annoyance, loudly saying things like "Why do they always put the students with me? They know I hate students." Even after becoming a nurse, there was an unspoken hierarchy that we newer nurses were expected to follow and that included things like who had to be on call, work weekends, and work night shifts.

Since I knew that Mr. Carl was in his eighties, I assumed that his wife, Ms. Mary, had thirty or more years of nursing experience on me, just like Travis did. He could tell I was anxious. "Don't worry," he assured me, "they'll love you."

Just then, a petite woman in her eighties came to the door, dressed in a hot pink tracksuit with her hair and makeup perfectly done. "Travis!" she exclaimed, hugging him. *Great,* I thought. *They're going to be so upset when they hear I'm replacing him.* Travis moved out of the way to introduce me. I could see the confusion on Mary's face as she looked back and forth between Travis and me.

"Yup, I got the management job," Travis told Mary before she could ask. "I'm going to pass Mr. Carl into Hadley's very capable hands."

Without missing a beat, Mary replied, "Well, we'll miss you, but we are happy for you. You all come on inside! The heat is stifling today. Let's get some sweet tea."

We walked into their charming cottage home, filled with plants, books, and natural light. I felt myself relax as Ms. Mary handed me a sweet tea. "I heard you're a nurse," I said tentatively.

She waved her hands as if to dismiss the idea. "Pediatrics,

honey. I don't know anything about hospice. As long as you tell me what you're doing before doing it, I will stay in my lane." She gave me a wink and a smile.

We followed Mary down a hallway and into a much darker bedroom just off the light-filled living room, where Mr. Carl was lying in a hospital bed. I was able to make out his features from the glow of the television.

"Honey, we got a new nurse," Mary cheerfully told her husband. Mr. Carl just grunted and turned the TV up louder. Travis chuckled to himself as he asked if he could turn the light on.

"No," Mr. Carl responded gruffly.

Travis did so anyway, apologizing and explaining that we would be in and out within ten minutes. Mr. Carl was clearly upset as Travis examined his skin, looking for any wounds that needed treatment. I watched on silently, trying to hide my reaction. While I was in no position to offer feedback, I felt that Travis shouldn't have asked for Mr. Carl's permission if he was just going to turn on the light in any case. It seemed to me that it was giving a false illusion of choice, which isn't good for someone in Mr. Carl's position, whose choices have already become so limited. I made a note to myself that if I were in a position like this in the future, I would instead explain what I was going to do and why, and assure the patient that I would finish as quickly as possible.

Finding no wounds to address, Travis gave Ms. Mary a quick rundown of the medications he would be refilling. She nodded in understanding.

Five minutes later, Travis and I were back outside in the hot sun. "He's grumpy. I should have warned you."

I shielded my eyes from the sun and silently looked toward

my car. For as much as working with other nurses showed me how I wanted to be with patients, sometimes it also showed me how I didn't want to be.

TWO DAYS LATER, I was back at Mr. Carl and Mary's door, but this time I was alone. Mr. Carl was my patient now, and I was ready to do things differently. It was obvious to me that Mr. Carl didn't like hospice—for very understandable reasons—and that he just wanted to be left alone to watch his shows without the nuisance. As a young and eager nurse, I was determined to change his mind.

When Ms. Mary opened the door, I realized with delight that she had on another tracksuit, this time royal blue, and her hair and makeup were once again perfectly done. I hoped to look as good as she did in fifty years. She waved me in and told me to go ahead into Mr. Carl's bedroom, and that she would be in in a minute.

Mr. Carl was in the same spot he'd been in when I last visited. Again, the room was lit only by the TV, and his white sheets were pulled up to his chin.

"Hey, Mr. Carl, can I come in?" I asked quietly, knocking softly on the bedroom door. He looked at me, confused for a moment, but nodded his head in silent agreement. Instead of turning on the light, I sat down on the chair at his bedside and asked what he was watching.

"Sports," he replied curtly.

I silently watched with him for a minute, noticing that he looked over at me every few seconds. "Don't you have stuff to do?" he finally asked.

"Yes, but I can wait for a commercial break. I'm in no rush."

He raised his eyebrows in obvious surprise, but didn't say anything and turned back to the TV.

Once the commercial came on, I asked if I could turn on the light to see his skin a little better. He nodded and I completed my assessment. As soon as I was done, I went to turn the light off, but he told me to keep it on. I obliged and sat back down to do my charting. After charting in silence for a few minutes, I noticed that my boyfriend Chris's favorite football team was playing.

"Oh, my boyfriend watched this last night!" I exclaimed. "He gets so excited about sports, but everything he tells me just goes over my head."

I saw Mr. Carl smile. It appeared that his hard shell was cracking a bit.

"I understand what a touchdown is, but what does a first down mean?" A little white lie wouldn't hurt.

"That's when they reach a point on the field and then get four more tries to keep going down the field toward a touchdown," he explained.

"*Oooh,* that makes sense!"

"Are you sure you're smart enough to be my nurse?" he asked with a chuckle.

I shrugged. "I guess you'll have to find out the hard way."

He laughed louder this time and Ms. Mary came rushing in, frantically asking what was wrong. When she realized we were laughing, her concern quickly melted away.

As we left Mr. Carl's room together, Ms. Mary put her arm around me and thanked me for making him smile. She said it had been months.

That night over dinner I eagerly told Chris about my new patient. He asked if I thought I would like the new assignment, then. "Yeah," I replied. "I feel like I'm making a difference."

"So proud of you," he said as he kissed my forehead and got up to clear our dishes from the table.

CHRIS WAS A PHYSICAL therapist whom I'd met at my previous job in the nursing home. When I'd first started working there, I noticed that his name came up a lot.

"Have you met the physical therapist yet?" Mrs. Stewart asked me as I changed the sheets from underneath her frail body.

"Not yet," I replied, distracted, checking her skin while I went along.

"He uses his lunch break to help me move my legs. My insurance said no more physical therapy visits so he does it for free."

I had never heard of a doctor doing something like that before. "That's amazing. He sounds amazing," I told her.

"He's great," she smiled, and winked.

I was taking a report from another nurse when I first met Chris. He was a handsome man in his thirties, and I could see his muscles even under his scrubs. He had a unique look, which I later came to understand was the result of his Greek Japanese heritage. The nurse introduced us and we both smiled at each other shyly. I briefly saw Ms. Morgan, a patient, stare at us before wheeling herself down the hall.

Later that day, Ms. Morgan rolled herself into the nurses' station while I sat there alone doing my charting.

"Are you single?" she asked.

"Yes," I answered, confused.

"You should talk to Chris more."

I laughed. "I'd love to, but I have no reason to go to his side of the building." The nursing home was set up in such a way that the residence and rehab were on two different sides of the building, separated by a cafeteria. The chances of us seeing each other outside of a random run-in at the cafeteria were slim.

Ms. Morgan knotted her eyebrows, clearly plotting something, before she quickly turned her wheelchair and rolled away. I peeked out from behind the doorframe to see where she was headed and watched as she stopped next to her friends—the Red Hat Society Ladies (a sorority-type association found in many nursing homes). As they talked and giggled, I noticed that they kept looking over at me every so often. I ducked my head and continued charting.

The next day, I was walking down the hallway when I saw Ms. Morgan lift her body out of her wheelchair and position herself on the ground. Extremely confused, I walked up to her. "Is everything okay, Ms. Morgan?"

"Oh honey, I'm afraid that I've fallen. I'll need to be evaluated by physical therapy. Will you be a dear and take me down there?"

My eyes widened as I looked at her, knowing she'd "fallen" intentionally. She put on an unconvincing show of grimacing in pain while her eyes danced with excitement. Unsure what else to do, I helped Ms. Morgan back into her wheelchair and wheeled her over to the therapy gym.

Chris quickly got up from his desk when he saw us.

"What's going on?" he asked as he knelt down next to Ms. Morgan.

"I'm such a klutz! I fell out of my chair and this sweet nurse was kind enough to help me up and bring me to you."

I didn't want to object so I only said, "It looks like you're in good hands, so I'll see you in a bit for your afternoon medications."

"Oh no! This will only take a minute. Why don't you stay so I don't have to wheel myself back so far?" Ms. Morgan said nonchalantly.

I shrugged and took a seat on the stack of blue gymnastics mats nearby as I watched Chris evaluate her. Only later did Chris tell me that it was obvious to him all along that nothing was wrong with Ms. Morgan. Still, he played along.

"Are you liking the new job?" he asked me while rotating Ms. Morgan's arm.

"It seems like everyone has worked here forever and all know each other so well. I feel a bit out of place as the newbie."

"I've worked here for four years and know everyone. I'd be happy to make introductions. Do you want to write your phone number down?" he asked, grabbing a notepad from his desk and handing it to me. I tried to hide my excitement as I wrote down my number and passed the notepad back.

Almost two years later, we were still going strong.

THREE DAYS AFTER MY initial solo visit to Mr. Carl, I was back again and feeling much more confident. Ms. Mary greeted me in her customary tracksuit, and waved me in to see my patient. I found him in his usual spot, but this time he was smiling.

"My boyfriend was so impressed with my football knowledge," I told him. "All thanks to you!"

"Oh, that's nothing," he replied. "We have a lot more work to do. Did you hear about Usain Bolt?"

"I have no idea what you are talking about," I said, laughing.

As I did my nursing assessment, Mr. Carl filled in all the details for me, explaining that Usain was a sprinter who had just taken the gold in two Olympic events for the third consecutive time. While I listened to Carl's heart and lungs, he said, "Don't tell your boyfriend I told you. Take the credit and see what he says."

I smiled and agreed.

Once I was back in my car and on my way to my next patient, I called Chris and told him what I'd heard about Usain.

"You heard about that?" he asked excitedly, rattling off obscure facts about Bolt's Olympic career. I happily let him tell me all about it as I drove the fifteen minutes to my next patient's home.

A few days later, I was pleased to report back to Mr. Carl how excited Chris was about my newfound interest in sports. We laughed together as Carl assured me it would be our secret. But behind my laughter, I felt a lump in my throat. I knew, by allowing a bond to grow between Carl and me, that I was setting myself up for heartbreak. I reminded myself to live for today, not the fears of tomorrow—a promise I had made to myself when I started working in hospice.

———

ONE DAY A FEW weeks later, Mr. Carl greeted me with a handwritten note. Confused, I opened it, and saw the news from the past few days written there in mostly legible cursive. "I started writing information down," he said. "Every time you leave, I remember something that I wanted to tell you. This way I won't forget."

"Perfect!" I replied. "Now I also won't forget."

Hours later, I picked Brody up from daycare and then sat in our driveway for a few moments before going in. Brody had fallen asleep on the way home, so while he slept I took the wrinkled paper out of my scrubs pocket and read it, smiling to myself. By this point, Carl's news updates had extended beyond just sports and also included current events and other newsworthy topics. He knew I was a single mom and never had time to sit down and watch or read the news, so he'd taken it upon himself to keep me informed. When I thanked him for doing this, Carl told me it gave him purpose and something to do. Folding the paper back up and placing it in my car's center console, I gently woke Brody and we walked into the house, where I shared the latest sports news with Chris over dinner. I silently thanked Mr. Carl for making me look way more knowledgeable than I was.

FOOTBALL SEASON CAME AND went, and the cold winter arrived.

One frigid Wednesday morning, I had a rare moment of downtime, sitting at my desk with a hot cup of coffee and talking to my co-worker.

As we were gossiping, Travis rushed in, interrupting our

laughter. "Hadley, it's Carl. Mary needs you." My co-worker looked at me sympathetically. She knew how much I adored Carl. I nodded and threw my heavy coat on as I hurried out of the office.

I could never have prepared myself for what happened next.

WALKING INTO CARL AND Mary's now-familiar home, I took off my coat and heard noises coming from the back of the house. Figuring it was Mary, I went into Carl's bedroom. As I stared at his empty hospital bed, my body filled with rage. Mr. Carl was dead and the funeral home had already come and taken him! Why hadn't Travis told me?

My rage turned to confusion when someone bumped me from behind. "Hey, Hadley," I heard. I spun around at the sound of Mr. Carl's voice.

I was momentarily blinded by a bright light. It wasn't *the* light that everyone talks about, but a heavy, black flashlight in Mr. Carl's hand. He walked past me as if on a mission.

Bewildered, I looked at Ms. Mary, who was walking right behind him, arms out to catch him if he were to tumble backward. She looked as confused as I felt.

"What's going on?" I whispered to her. "I've never seen him out of bed. I didn't think he could walk!"

"Me neither," she panic-whispered back to me.

"How long has this been going on?"

"At least an hour. He won't talk to me. He just walks around the house with this flashlight, looking behind curtains and in small spaces. I was hoping *you* could tell me what is going on."

Wide-eyed, I shook my head no.

I turned back to Mr. Carl, who was now on his hands and knees looking under his hospital bed. "Whatcha doing?" I asked, trying to sound as casual as possible, though I could hear my voice wavering.

"I'm playing hide-and-seek with Anna," he replied, as if it was the most obvious thing in the world. Having never heard of Anna before, I turned toward Ms. Mary to ask and saw that her eyes had filled with tears and her hands were clutched to her heart. After taking a moment to compose herself, she explained, "Anna is our baby girl. She drowned when she was two years old. Carl blamed himself. It wasn't anyone's fault, but he never forgave himself for not being there to save her."

Chills ran up and down my spine as I processed this information. I had no idea what to say or do. And then the voice of one of my favorite nursing school instructors popped into my head: *Meet them where they are.*

But the question was: Where was Carl? It seemed as if he was in two places at once—physically, he was here in this room with Mary and me; emotionally and mentally, he seemed very much to be somewhere else, with Anna. In the time since Ms. Glenda had passed, I'd seen this end-of-life visitation with a few other patients as well. The phenomenon seemed less and less unexpected and more and more natural to me— but I'd never seen a patient be visited by a child. And this was compounded by the fact that, after several months together, I hadn't realized until this very moment that Carl and Mary

ever had a child, nor had I ever seen Carl move from his bed—
and yet here he was, spry as could be.

Okay, I thought, *I can do this.* I slowly turned back to Mr.
Carl, who was now in the bathroom, rummaging through the
linen closet.

"What can I do to help you find her?" I asked him.

He looked directly at me with tears in his eyes and said, "I
know where she is."

"You do?"

"Yes, but I can't get to her yet. I think I will soon, though.
That's what my mom said."

"You're seeing your mom too?" I asked.

"Yes," he replied matter-of-factly.

"What should we do now?"

"I guess lie down." He shrugged.

I nodded and gently led Carl back to his hospital bed.

WITH CARL SETTLED, Ms. Mary and I hugged and I instructed her to call if she needed us during the night. I walked
out the front door and into the cold air just as the sun was
setting, coloring the world in a breathtaking array of reds, or-
anges, and purples. I took a minute to admire the sky and was
momentarily distracted by a bluebird who was perched on the
branch of a nearby tree, still and watching me with a steady
gaze. I briefly wondered if it was Anna before pushing the
thought out of my head. I was being silly. This was all just a
coincidence. Or a hallucination. Or something like that.

I got into my car, cranked up the heat, and dialed the number of our hospice physician, Dr. Kumar. I always enjoyed

speaking with him because he was both extremely smart and very approachable, and always willing to talk. He was very different from any other physician I'd ever worked with—much more laid-back, and very trusting of the nurses he worked with.

"Hey, what's going on?" he answered.

"Are you busy right now? It's not an emergency."

I watched the bluebird through my windshield, still perched and unmoving, and still staring directly at me. So strange.

"Nope. Whatcha got?"

"I wanted to update you on Mr. Carl. He walked today. I have never seen him walk before."

"Oh, okay. The surge," Dr. Kumar replied, sounding not at all surprised, and almost distracted.

"Uh, the what?"

"The surge of energy almost everyone gets before dying," he said, as if this was a well-known medical fact. I now know that the surge is a common occurrence. Often, loved ones who witness it think that the patient is somehow miraculously in the process of recovering. But to those in the know, it's a sign that death is imminent and will likely occur within the next few days.

"I guess so," I replied, still unaware of this fact. "I'm still new to this. He was also seeing his deceased mother and child."

"Was it distressing for him?"

"No, he was calm."

"He'll probably pass soon," Dr. Kumar said, just as the bluebird flew away from the branch.

"Did you not hear me?" I exclaimed. "He was walking! He is getting better. His vital signs were all normal. He isn't dying."

"You'll see, Hadley," Dr. Kumar said quietly, and we hung up the phone.

I was uneasy after the day's events. When I finally forced myself to go to bed, I dreamed all night of a little blond girl with pigtails, running through wildflowers with bluebirds happily flying alongside her. I woke up feeling like I hadn't slept for a moment.

THE NEXT DAY, I showed up at Mr. Carl's home like I did every Tuesday morning, unsure of what I would find. Mr. Carl was back in his bed with Ms. Mary at his side.

"He's only staying awake for a few minutes at a time," she told me.

Just then, Mr. Carl opened his eyes and smiled at me. "Hey, there's my favorite nurse." He was weak, barely able to keep his eyes open or talk at his usual pace.

"There's my favorite patient," I replied. It was true. Although I was working with about twelve patients by this point, I felt a unique bond with Carl and Mary. I'm sure that some of it was because he remained in hospice for several months—but it was more than that too. I felt bonded to and at ease with them. "You had a big day yesterday," I said softly. "As soon as I'm done with my assessment I'll let you rest."

I listened to Carl's heart and lungs, as I had done so many times before.

"Thank you," he said.

"For what?"

"For giving me something to look forward to instead of death." I felt hot tears on my cheeks and flushed with embarrassment. "I'm gonna miss you, kid," he said, barely able to keep his eyes open at this point.

"I'm gonna miss you too, Mr. Carl," I replied, unable to see through my tears.

As Ms. Mary walked me out, she asked me how much longer I thought he had left.

"I don't really know, to be honest," I answered, trying to compose myself.

I CRAWLED INTO BED with a heavy heart that night. I wasn't ready for Mr. Carl to pass. He had become like a grandfather to me. I tried scrolling through Instagram to distract myself, but it didn't help much. After drifting off to sleep sometime around 10:00 P.M., I was abruptly woken up by my cell phone ringing at 4:00 A.M. It was the primary on-call nurse.

"Hadley, I am so sorry. I'm across town helping a patient in pain and I just got a call from Mr. Carl's wife that sounded urgent. She needs someone to come to their home. Can you please go?" Although I was the backup nurse that night, after nearly a year in hospice I had yet to receive a call to visit a patient at night. Because we had two night-shift nurses as well, backups were only called in when they were both busy, which was unlikely.

"Of course," I replied and hung up.

"Who was that? I thought you weren't on call," Chris said groggily.

"Mr. Carl needs me," I told him, already getting out of bed. "I'm on backup, and I've never been called before."

Chris looked at me sympathetically. "Then you better get going," he said. "I've got Brody handled. Take all the time you need."

I kissed him goodbye and headed out the door.

My chest felt heavy as I drove to Carl and Mary's home. I replayed my first meeting with Mr. Carl, and remembered all of the sports facts he'd shared with me over the months, and the many sweet teas I had drunk while talking to him and Mary. I also thought about his final words to me yesterday morning.

When I arrived at their home, something felt different. I timidly walked toward his bedroom, where Ms. Mary met me outside the door.

"He's gone," she said, almost sympathetically, as if to ease the blow.

"Okay," I breathed with a heavy sigh. I immediately apologized, embarrassed, realizing that this was Mary's loss and I needed to be strong for her.

Mary and I walked into the bedroom together, which was completely dark without the glow from the TV. I turned on a lamp and stared down at Mr. Carl's lifeless body. I placed my stethoscope on his chest as I had done so many times before, but this time there was no familiar, rhythmic *thump, thump, thump* in my ears. I wasn't looking down at his smiling, weathered face. Not this time. This time there was silence. Emptiness.

I couldn't stop the tears from coming and was barely able to croak out, "Time of death: 4:47 A.M." I looked up and my tear-filled eyes met Ms. Mary's. She walked over and hugged me as I cried harder.

"I'm sorry, I'm so sorry. I'm supposed to be comforting you," I said through my sobs. She pulled back to look at me and firmly said, "We are comforting each other. Never apologize. We both love you so much. God put you in our lives. We both know this."

I nodded in silence, unable to speak as the tears continued to flow. As I sank into Mary, I thought back to how intimidated I'd been by her at first. It seemed funny now, when all I'd ever felt from her was love and acceptance, not to mention her complete confidence in my abilities. After a few minutes, I composed myself.

"What now?" she asked.

"I have to call the funeral home."

Mary sighed and nodded.

After I made the call, Ms. Mary and I dressed Mr. Carl in the navy suit he wanted to leave his home in. Together we pulled on his suit jacket, a difficult feat, and I grabbed his cherry-red tie from the chair that I had sat in so many times before. I handed the tie to Mary. "I don't know how to tie a tie."

She took the tie back from me and chuckled. "I don't either." All of a sudden, her chuckles turned into a full-on belly laugh. "I just know that if he was here right now, he would ask how he can trust us with patients' lives if we can't even tie a tie."

I began laughing too, and we didn't stop until the doorbell rang. I went to answer the door with a smile still on my face, Ms. Mary's laughter echoing behind me. I'm sure the funeral home workers thought we were a little crazy.

As they placed Mr. Carl onto the gurney and pulled the white sheet over him, Ms. Mary stopped them, suddenly remembering something.

"Socks!" she said. "He has to wear socks!" I looked at her. "Anna. He put socks on her before they took her away when she passed. He said he didn't want her feet to get cold."

I nodded in understanding and handed the tie and socks to the funeral home workers.

Before they left, they needed my signature, a common procedure. I realized I didn't have a pen on me, and not wanting to burden Ms. Mary, I walked out to my car to grab one. As I searched my car for a pen, I felt my hand touch a wad of paper. Confused, I pulled it out and realized I was holding the first note Mr. Carl had ever written me, so many months before. I sighed heavily as I touched his handwriting.

I quickly walked back inside to give the waiting funeral home workers my signature. I held the front door open for them and leaned my head against the doorframe to watch them take Mr. Carl away.

As they wheeled him down the driveway and into the waiting hearse, I heard chirping nearby and looked up at a nearby tree, where I saw a bluebird. It happily chirped a few times and then began flapping its wings. I watched in awe as the bird flew directly alongside the hearse.

I smiled to myself with tears in my eyes, and whispered, "Take good care of your daddy for me, Anna."

Sue

THE FALL AFTER CARL DIED, I WAS ASSIGNED TO MS. Sue, a patient who had been dealing with chronic obstructive pulmonary disease (COPD), which is actually a range of diseases that make the patient's breathing labored; taking even a few steps across the room can cause them to feel like they've run a marathon and are struggling for air.

I first met Ms. Sue on a brisk autumn morning. I was warmly welcomed into her home by her son, Fred, who looked like he wasn't a day over fifty, although I figured he must be older given that his mother was ninety-eight. His wife, Leanne, was right behind him and equally friendly.

After some initial pleasantries, Fred launched in: "We want to warn you, she's feisty and very strong-willed. She's had COPD for years, but the other night it got so bad that we called 911. Once she was in the emergency room and breathing well again, she refused any treatment or further testing. So, of course, the doctor recommended hospice."

"That makes sense. I can't wait to meet her. I'm used to

feisty and strong-willed!" I replied confidently. Although I still had a lot to learn, by this point I had treated several patients on my own, and COPD is a common disease in the hospice world, so I'd worked with it before.

As we made our way into the next room, I saw Ms. Sue sitting in a large, comfy-looking chair that practically swallowed her whole. She couldn't have weighed more than ninety pounds and her bones were visible, an unfortunate side effect of her disease.

I greeted Ms. Sue with my usual peppy "Hi! I'm Hadley! It's so nice to meet you!"

"I don't see what the point of *you* is," she replied, exasperated.

I was taken aback. *What was my point?* It took me what felt like a lifetime to form a coherent thought but I finally responded, "I'm here to make you comfortable."

"I feel fine," she said curtly.

I looked to her son for help.

"Mom, she's with hospice," Fred cut in. "Remember, Dr. Smith said she would come so you don't have to go to the emergency room anymore."

"I know that," Ms. Sue replied to her son sharply, then added, "I didn't ask you to be here."

I snuck a look over at Fred, but he didn't seem affected by his mom's comment. It was a fine line to walk between taking control of a situation and not offending vulnerable patients and their families, and I was desperate to get this right. I remained silent, uncertain how to respond. After several seconds, Ms. Sue finally turned to me and said, "You can do what you need to, but I don't know if I will keep you as my nurse."

Relieved, I began filling out the necessary paperwork to admit her onto hospice services. When I finished, I suggested I return the next day for a normal visit. I also explained that hospice nurses are available 24/7, but I wouldn't necessarily be the one on call at any given time.

"Would it be okay for me to come back tomorrow, or would you prefer a different nurse?" I asked.

Sue replied with a sigh, then said, "I guess so. Come tomorrow and we will take it day by day."

Fred smiled and rolled his eyes. As he walked me out, he said, "I think she likes you."

I tried to hide how crazy I thought he was.

THE NEXT DAY, I made my normal visit to Ms. Sue, checking her blood pressure, pulse, respirations, and temperature. I examined her skin for any pressure sores or bruises. I asked about her bowel movements, if she had any side effects from her medications, and how her eating and sleeping were. She answered each question curtly, and as I charted she watched golf on TV, not speaking much.

Our visits continued like this, twice a week for a month, until one day Ms. Sue turned the volume down on the TV and looked at me. "Why do you stay so long after you finish everything?" she asked. "You could probably be in and out of here in fifteen minutes."

"The company I work for requires me to stay for at least

thirty minutes, but they prefer that I stay for forty-five." Sue was right—sometimes there wasn't anything to do or take care of for that amount of time, which meant that I got to sit down and listen to my patients' stories, which I loved.

"You know you could just sit in your car for fifteen minutes and no one would know the difference. No one listens to us old biddies, anyway. They all think I'm confused just because I'm older than dirt."

I chuckled before saying, "I'm a single mom. I can't risk losing my job." This was a detail I didn't often share with my patients. There was a general rule in my company not to share our private lives. One time a family member called our manager saying they felt as if the nurse's problems were being put on them. It's true that all of the families we're dealing with have a lot on their plate, and they certainly don't need any more stress added to their load. And it's also true that sometimes we hospice nurses spend a significant period of time with patients and their families and develop a relationship with them, and it feels strange *not* to share. I tried to walk the line between following the rules and connecting with patients. And I definitely wanted to connect with Ms. Sue after weeks of silence.

It didn't work, though. Instead of continuing the conversation, she nodded and turned the volume back up.

I guessed we were going back to not talking.

ON MY NEXT VISIT, Ms. Sue was in her usual spot. Her white hair was perfectly curled as always, and her housedress matched her slippers. But this time, she started talking before I could even sit down.

"Slept six hours. Pooped this morning. Didn't want to eat breakfast. Last meal was dinner last night, and I ate it all. My sweater is already off, so you can take my blood pressure and look at my skin."

I quickly pulled out my tablet to write everything down. After I plugged in all the information, I pulled out my stethoscope. When I finished, I placed my tablet down to indicate that I was done.

"You still have a lot of time left, right?" she asked.

"Yes, at least twenty minutes."

"Can you water my plants?"

This wasn't a typical nursing task; this more general sort of help usually fell to nursing aides, but I didn't see why I couldn't assist. "Sure!" I replied enthusiastically. Ms. Sue directed me to the watering can. As I filled it up, I looked at the pictures on her wall. There was a wedding portrait of a much younger Ms. Sue, still tiny, but being swallowed by a ginormous wedding dress rather than a chair, and standing next to a man in military uniform. As I looked around, I noticed that this same man—clearly her husband—was all over the walls, dressed in uniform in almost every picture.

Ms. Sue pointed at each plant and told me when to start and stop watering. Some plants needed lots of water and others only needed a few drops. I had to fill the watering can back up a few times before I finished.

"Can you do this once a week?"

"Of course," I agreed enthusiastically. At least she was finally talking to me.

"Good. I'll keep you as my nurse if you can actually make yourself useful. Next time, bring in the mail with you."

"Yes ma'am," I said, with a big smile. Honestly, it was kind of nice to do something outside of my normal routine.

ON MY NEXT VISIT, I placed Ms. Sue's mail on the table and she nodded in acknowledgment, which was the extent of her gratitude. As she'd done on the previous visit, she rattled off her answers to my usual questions, letting me know she'd slept, pooped, and eaten. After completing my assessment, I put my tablet into my bag to indicate that I was ready for my next assignment.

"There's laundry on the bed. Can you fold worth a shit?"

I pondered my laundry-folding skills for a minute before slowly nodding my head. "My mom taught me. I think I do it correctly."

With that, Sue pointed her slender, red-manicured finger in the direction of her bedroom. Her all-white bed was perfectly made, adorned with a delicate lace bed skirt with a scalloped edge. It was beautiful. I noticed another wedding picture on her bedside table.

When I returned to the living room with the laundry in tow, I plopped down on the floor to begin folding, and decided to try my luck. "I saw your wedding pictures. They are beautiful. How long were you married for?"

"Not long enough," she replied, not taking her eyes off the TV. "He died in his late twenties. War."

"Your son said he had three siblings. Did you remarry?" I asked, as I folded one of her silky undershirts. Ms. Sue turned off the TV and faced me.

"You're nosy."

I worried that I had upset her. "Sorry, I just want to learn about you," I said, not taking my eyes off the shirt in my lap.

"No one ever asks about me. It's always just 'Take this medication,' 'Go to this doctor's appointment,'" she said while gazing out the window, seemingly deep in thought.

I kept quiet and continued folding. After about a minute, she looked at me and started talking. "I never remarried. We got married when I was sixteen. My parents had known him since he was born. He was the absolute love of my life. I was pregnant with our fourth, Fred, when he was drafted. I remember kissing him, his hand on my large belly, and knowing that I'd never see him again."

I looked up from my folding as Sue said that last line. Her lips were pursed, her attention inward; she looked as if she was watching a memory. "I can't even imagine . . ." I said, trailing off, unsure if that was an appropriate thing to say.

"Oh, honey, that's not how you fold. Give me that. Watch," she said suddenly, grabbing the shirt from my hands. I watched as Ms. Sue folded the shirt perfectly, but I was distracted by what she'd shared with me. I wanted to hear more.

THE NEXT TIME I came to visit, Sue was having more difficulty than usual breathing. It was noticeable as soon as I saw her.

"How long have you been breathing like this?" I asked.

"It's been since yesterday, but I'm totally fine."

I pulled out my stethoscope, hearing the wheezing, like a high-pitched whistle, as soon as I placed it on her chest. I pulled out my pulse oximeter, a small machine that clips on the patient's finger to measure the amount of oxygen in their blood, and placed it on Sue's cold finger: 87% popped up. I breathed a sigh of relief that her oxygen wasn't too bad. But my relief quickly turned to panic when I realized that she was having symptoms I didn't know how to treat—extreme shortness of breath, like if you imagine a fish that's jumped out of water and is unable to get back in.

I excused myself to call the doctor. I was trying to remain calm, but Ms. Sue was turning blue and I was worried she was going to die if I didn't take action quickly.

"What should I do?" I asked Dr. Kumar frantically.

"Is she in any pain? Is she uncomfortable at all?"

"No, she said she's not in any pain. She says she's fine, but I can't just let her have labored breathing and wheezing!"

"You can," he replied calmly. "I understand nursing school only taught you to treat, treat, treat. In this case, that would mean sticking her with a large needle, drawing tons of blood, admitting her to the hospital, giving her tons of medications, and who knows what else. She doesn't want that. All she wants is to be at home and comfortable. I know it's against what you've been taught, but you're doing what you're supposed to be doing. She is at home and she's comfortable."

I nodded, letting Dr. Kumar's words sink in. Maybe sometimes people didn't need more—maybe, sometimes, they needed . . . less. Maybe sometimes all they needed was a little bit of comfort.

OF COURSE, DR. KUMAR hadn't told me anything that I didn't already know about the function of hospice, but until that moment I hadn't realized how deeply ingrained in me it was to always treat: more labs, more medications, more scans. Nursing school has everything to do with learning how to heal patients—or at least try to—and little to do with how to comfort them.

In my second year of nursing school, four people from my class were selected to do a one-year internship at a local hospital, where we were paid to shadow nurses full-time during the summer and part-time during the school year. I was overjoyed to be selected for the program.

Each morning, the three other interns and I clocked in, and then looked at the board for our predetermined assignments.

"Med/Surg," I groaned one day early on in my internship. It was my least favorite floor.

"ICU for me," my friend Summer replied. "Heather got labor and delivery again." We both wanted to be labor and delivery nurses.

"Hey, you with me today?" a middle-aged nurse with her hair in a low ponytail said, gesturing toward me as she clocked in. Her name was Theresa, and she worked in the emergency department. I'd worked one shift with her last week and really liked her.

"I wish! Med/Surg," I replied, pointing at the board in front of us.

"Oh no, don't go there. You'll learn more with me today. Come on." As I watched Theresa speed-walk toward the emergency department, I turned to Summer, who shrugged. I shrugged back and waved goodbye as I jogged to catch up to Theresa.

"I don't think my manager will be okay with this," I said as I struggled to keep up with her.

"Blame it on me. I've worked here longer than your manager. She won't say anything to me." Theresa scanned her badge to enter the locked emergency department. Before I could even put my belongings down, she was rushing into room eight.

"Theresa, I need Epi now," the scrub-clad doctor in the room called over his shoulder. I could see the sweat on his brow as he tried to bring his patient back to life. Theresa was already rifling through the drawer on the crash cart, a utility cart that has all of the tools and medicine you might need if a patient is crashing.

She waved me over. "Find the Epi," she told me calmly.

I started to sweat as I searched, but couldn't find it. "I'll just watch. I'm not ready," I told her, stepping back, overwhelmed.

Theresa grabbed the epinephrine, which was on the cart just as she said it would be, and handed it to the nurse nearest the patient. "You're doing the next task," she commanded. I felt like I was going to pass out.

"We need access in the other arm," someone in the room said. Theresa squeezed my shoulder before gathering the supplies to place an IV in the lifeless patient's arm. She shoved the supplies at me as I shook my head in protest.

"Look, you can either do it now while I'm here to help or you can do it one day by yourself." I nodded and began unpacking the supplies with shaky hands, scared that I would miss the vein with all these people watching. Thankfully, Theresa guided my hand and I got it in successfully on my first try.

The pride and accomplishment I felt lasted about a minute before the doctor made an announcement.

"He's gone. I'm calling it. Time of death: 7:17." Everyone stopped what they were doing and began to file out of the room.

The only people left were Theresa, the patient, and me. She logged onto the computer by the bed while I stared at the dead man. He looked horrible. His skin was tinted blue, his clothes were ripped away from his body, a tube extended from his mouth, and blood stained the sheets. Trash was littered on the floor around him—medication vials, gauze, and packaging. I didn't know what had happened to him, what his name was, or how old he was.

I heard the sliding glass door open behind me and turned to see a petite woman come in, her face stained with mascara from her tears. It was clear that she was close to the deceased patient, but I didn't know how.

"I'm so sorry," I said to the woman, feeling the need to console her.

"Take your time and let someone know when you're done," Theresa said to her as she motioned for me to follow.

"We don't have time to console," Theresa told me. "We have three other patients that need us right now."

Despite what Theresa had said, I paused. I could hear the woman crying through the door—this felt wrong.

But Theresa was right that every other patient needed us too. We didn't take any breaks that day as we cared for what felt like hundreds of patients, each of whom was having the worst day of their life. Despite being much older than me,

Theresa never seemed to tire physically or mentally. She was able to go from patient to patient without getting emotionally invested. I, on the other hand, found myself still thinking of the last patient while listening to the next patient's traumatic story. I envied Theresa's ability to disconnect and wanted to emulate her dispassionate demeanor. She was highly respected by the other nurses and doctors, and I wanted to be respected too.

I spent most of that summer shadowing Theresa, learning everything I could from her. I got better at being able to emotionally disconnect and focus on the tasks at hand.

One day, we were treating a patient with diabetes and foot pain. "The surgeon should be coming to see you within the hour," Theresa said to him.

"He doesn't need to do that. I won't be getting surgery," the patient replied. I looked at the man's foot. It was evident that he needed surgery, and I didn't understand why he was refusing it.

"You'll die without it," Theresa said nonchalantly, never taking her eyes off the screen where she was reviewing the patient's chart.

"God will save me if I'm meant to live."

"All righty, then." Theresa shrugged, exiting the room while I followed closely behind her.

"Stupid," she said to me as we walked down the hall.

"I agree that he should get surgery, but do you not believe him?" I asked her.

"No, honey. I don't know anyone who works in the emergency department that does. A higher power that allows what we see to happen isn't someone I want to spend eternity with."

I felt the pull between how I had been raised and what I was experiencing. Everyone seemed to have different ideas about God and religion and what it all meant. How was I supposed to know who was right and who was wrong? Growing up, I was told to lean on God and never question his plan—just like this man in the ER was—but I understood where Theresa was coming from as well. In the short amount of time I had spent in the ER, which paled in comparison to the years she had spent working there, I had also seen some true horrors.

But now, in hospice, I was seeing something totally different. Patients from all different religious and non-religious backgrounds were having spiritual encounters that I couldn't ignore. Patients whom I had the opportunity to get to know, love, and trust. I was coming to realize that it wasn't as black and white as I had previously thought it was—there was certainly an in-between.

I SHOOK MY HEAD, as if to shake away all of the lessons I'd learned in my time as a nursing intern in the ER, when I strove to put firm boundaries around what I offered patients in their time of need—which was treatment, not comfort. I thought briefly about how Theresa might react to this conversation with Dr. Kumar and expected there would be some eye-rolling involved.

"So, I just do . . . nothing?" I finally replied to Dr. Kumar.

"No, you call her family and give them an update. You get her favorite foods and let her do her favorite things. You ask her again if she's comfortable and when she isn't you call me back so we can make sure she is, and you keep doing that until she is happy. What you are doing is important, even if society doesn't always see that."

Dr. Kumar and I said our goodbyes and hung up. From that moment on, I started thinking differently about patient care. I started to reframe my work with the understanding that sometimes doing "nothing" (as I would have thought of it in nursing school and my previous jobs) was doing something. It was being there, offering comfort and solidarity—and that mattered. A lot. This was a new realization for me because, even though I'd been in hospice for a year and a half by this point and understood that my job wasn't to save my patients, I was still always offering something, usually as a means of alleviating pain. In this instance, though, there was truly nothing to do but to *be* with Ms. Sue.

When I returned to Sue, I let her know that the doctor's only concern was her comfort.

"Oh, that makes me feel so much better. I was so worried that you were calling an ambulance to come whisk me away," she said. The relief was obvious in her voice. I smiled, feeling like I had made the right choice.

"Once you finish up, can you make me a sandwich?" she asked.

"Of course!" I responded cheerfully, hearing Dr. Kumar's voice in my head. But first I quickly completed my assessment, which included asking Ms. Sue if she was sure she was comfortable and pain-free at least three more times. She was still short of breath, but adamant that she was used to it and did not want any treatment. I then put my tablet away and asked Ms. Sue to tell me exactly what kind of sandwich she wanted. I walked to the kitchen, determined to make the best turkey-and-Swiss-with-mayo-and-tomato sandwich ever. I searched her pantry for the bread. "Do you have another loaf of bread? This one's expired," I called out.

"Is there mold on it?" Sue yelled back.

I pulled out a few slices with my gloved hands, and turned them over to check. "No mold, but I still think I should use a new loaf."

"Honey, use that bread and once you bring my sandwich over, I've got a thing or two to tell ya," she said.

I obliged, finishing up her sandwich and carefully placing it on one of her dainty white plates. As Ms. Sue took small bites of her lunch, she began to tell me about growing up during the Great Depression and how, to this day, as a result of that experience, she never wasted food. She also told me about how she couldn't attend school sometimes because she had to help support her family by working. After the Depression, when Sue was in her twenties, she went on to become a teacher.

Once she finished her sandwich, Sue must have decided that story time was over. As she handed me her empty plate, Ms. Sue told me it was time for me to get going. I cleaned off her plate and called out my goodbye, but didn't get a response.

MY NEXT VISIT WAS a plant-watering day. When I arrived, Sue wasn't in her usual housedress and slippers, but was instead wearing a matching skirt and jacket with tights and low heels.

"Wow, look at you! Big plans?"

"Well, nothing is a big deal at my age, but I do have an event at the church I'm quite excited about. When you get to be my age, making your face known to the Lord becomes more and more important."

"Have you always been religious?" I asked her.

"Yes, I've always found comfort in my religion, especially when my husband died. What about you, dear? You ask an awful lot of questions about me."

I let the watering can hang by my side for a moment as I pondered the question, still so unsure about the answer. "I was raised very religious. I would say . . . I'm still trying to figure it all out. I wish I knew."

"I think there are more people out there that agree with you than would care to admit. I guess I'll learn the truth soon, though."

"Are you scared?" I asked before I could process what I was asking.

"No," she said simply. I watered the plants and completed my assessment, preoccupied with the thought of how strange it must feel to know you'll die soon, and how happy I was that Sue found comfort in her beliefs.

IT HAD BEEN A long time since I'd felt what Sue did, but our discussion made me think about what a powerful sense of comfort the church had offered me in those early days of my pregnancy, when I was scared and confused.

I had just returned home for the summer after my freshman year of college, and I had a stomach bug that I didn't seem able to shake. Finally, my mom had enough of hearing me vomit up bile. "That's it! We're going to immediate care," she told me.

When we arrived, I took a seat in the lobby to fill out the health questionnaire. As I stared at the question asking when my last period was, I started to panic. My periods had always been irregular, but I couldn't recall having one the month prior or even the month before that. I left the space blank as another wave of nausea washed over me.

In the exam room, a tall nurse with hot pink scrubs and curly hair piled on top of her head walked in with a clear cup in her hand.

"All right, honey, first things first: pregnancy test."

I avoided eye contact with my mom as I exited the room to the bathroom.

When I returned, my mom looked at me. "Is there a chance?" she asked.

"No, I'm not pregnant," I said.

Almost as if on cue, the nurse walked back in and loudly announced, "You're pregnant."

I felt my eyes well up with tears as my mom started rubbing my back.

The nurse comforted me as she wrote on her clipboard. "Now, baby, don't cry," she said. "You have options. Don't let anyone tell you that you don't. This is your body, okay?"

I nodded, and then my mom and I walked out of the office and into the bright sun. The only thing my mom said to me on the ride home was, "I won't judge you and I won't push my personal beliefs on you. If you want to keep it, I'll love it. If you don't want to, I'll take that secret to the grave."

When we got home, I went straight upstairs to my childhood bedroom, where I lay on my bed and looked out the window. Rows of beach houses just like ours lined the street. Rows of homes with families that I aspired to be like. Families that were started when two people fell in love in college, graduated, got married, had children, and bought their perfect little home near the beach.

I can still have that, I told myself. *I can get an abortion and no one will ever know.* I began searching for abortion clinics near me. I found the closest one and read up on the process, deciding that I would book an appointment on Monday. I wrote the phone number down on a piece of paper and placed it in my nightstand drawer, not wanting my mom to see. I knew I couldn't have her come to the appointment with me; I felt too much shame.

The next morning, the sun was peeking through my window when I woke up. I went into the bathroom and stripped down to take a shower. As I looked in the mirror, I imagined a baby in my belly. It was such a foreign concept, it didn't even feel real. As I walked downstairs, I saw my mom getting out her car keys to go to church. She normally spent all morning and afternoon at church on Sundays, and I really didn't want to be alone with my thoughts. I asked her if I could go with her. By this point, I had spent many years disassociating while in church and not taking any of it seriously, so I knew this mass wouldn't sway me from what I intended to do. I just didn't want to be alone. I could tell my mom was surprised by my request, but she just nodded. She probably thought if I was willing to go to church, I was leaning toward keeping the baby—but I wasn't.

We arrived at the church my mom had started going to

after she divorced my dad when I was seventeen, one I had never been to before. I thought that it was the most beautiful church I had ever seen. It was made of glass and, if you listened closely, you could hear the ocean waves lapping onto the shore nearby. We found a seat near the back and sang along to the hymns. I was distracted, bored, and wondered why I had come.

Finally the priest, Father Tom, an older man wearing silky robes, raised his hands to the sky, holding a Bible in one hand and a notebook in the other. After a few moments, he placed both down on the podium in front of him.

He stared down at the open books in complete silence, then finally closed the notebook and began speaking. "I had a sermon planned for today. I spent an entire day writing it, but God is telling me I have someone here to speak to."

I rolled my eyes, thinking this was just a cheap way to keep people's attention.

"God's plan can sometimes feel confusing," he began. "Many times we might find ourselves saying, *Why me, God? Or, Why couldn't you have given me their life instead? It looks so much easier.*"

Well, that does apply to me, I thought, *but I'm sure it applies to half the people in this room as well.*

"On my way inside, I was stopped by a couple with two children," he continued. "They asked me to take their picture, and as I was taking it I was spoken to. Someone in here yearns for this couple's life. They want the white picket fence—to graduate college and get married, have two kids, and live happily ever after. But that's not what God needs them for."

I watched my mom out of the corner of my eye as he spoke,

but she never took her eyes off of Father Tom. I began picking at my chipped fingernail polish.

"You're going to have to give up your ideal life in order to live the life planned for you. You're going to have to give up your sorority, your college life, and this path you're currently on."

I blatantly looked at my mom this time, only to see that her mouth was hanging open in shock. I was shocked too, because now this was very specific to my situation. But as I glanced around the room, I saw many girls my age.

"You need to have this baby," he continued. *All right, what is going on?!* I wondered. This was way too close to home. I glared at my mom, thinking she had somehow orchestrated this, but she swears to this day that she never said a word to anyone in the church and did not have a clue that I would come with her that morning.

"Life is not going to be easy at first, but this is the life planned for you and it will be worth it," Father Tom finished.

As my mom and I walked out of the church, I felt more confused than ever. We rode home in silence, and I spent every waking moment between then and Monday agonizing over my choice.

On Monday morning, I held the phone number of the abortion clinic in my hands, but I couldn't bring myself to call. What if Father Tom was right? What if this was the path for me? I knew life wouldn't be easy if I kept the baby—and it certainly wouldn't be the life I had imagined.

The days turned into weeks, and I never called the clinic. My mom and I didn't talk about it until one day when she told me I needed to make a doctor's appointment. I was starting to show, and the window for me to decide was rapidly closing.

As I called the ob-gyn for a prenatal appointment, my fate seemed sealed. In that moment, I felt like everything was going to be okay. Somehow, in the place I least expected it, I had found comfort.

AS TIME HAS PASSED, I've found it to be generally true in life that, in the end, things are usually okay. Sometimes it just takes a lot of hard work and uncertainty to get there. That seemed to be proving the case in my situation with Sue too. After working with her for a few months, I found out that on the days when I was unavailable, Ms. Sue would simply refuse care—in her mind, it was me or nobody, and if I couldn't come to her house she would simply remain in pain. While I certainly didn't want Ms. Sue to be in pain, it also bolstered my sense of confidence to have won the trust of this woman who had been so skeptical of me and the healthcare field in general. It let me know that she knew I really saw her and was invested in her. It felt like validation that I was on the right path, and it also reinforced what Dr. Kumar had told me— that sometimes just being there and offering a measure of comfort wasn't only enough—it was everything.

AS I CONTINUED TO care for Ms. Sue, she told me all about her life. My favorite stories were from when she traveled the world. She and her best friend were teachers for many years, and as soon as they had saved up enough money, they quit their jobs and traveled together for two years. When I asked Sue how she felt about leaving her kids behind she told me, "They got postcards and I got to see the Eiffel Tower."

Sue was quick and spunky, especially for someone of her age and in her condition. I grew to understand that what I had at first thought to be coldness was actually a mixture of a quirky sense of humor and a defensive response to feeling discarded or left behind.

Sue helped me understand how isolating growing old can be. She wasn't afraid of death, and faith was a big part of this; but her attitude was also based on the fact that, as she put it, "all of my friends are dead."

"Are you sure?" I finally asked her.

As it turned out, Sue wasn't *really* sure about that. When I probed, I found out that Sue had never used the internet. So, during one of my visits, she had me sit with her and Google all of her friends to confirm that they were, in fact, dead. In the cases where the internet didn't have an answer, Sue asked me to search for her friends' children so that she could get on the phone and ask if they were dead (and yes, that's exactly how Sue ever-so-delicately phrased it).

And one of Sue's friends wasn't dead, after all—and not just any friend, but the fellow teacher whom she'd traveled the world with. The two of them started writing letters back and forth, which were hilarious. They were almost like teenagers complaining about their parents, except these two were complaining about their kids. Sue wrote about how her family had moved her down to Florida, and her friend complained about how hers stuck her in a nursing home.

Those letters and that connection meant a lot to Sue, and it was beautiful to see her life expand. While I was never trained for it in nursing school, I know that watering Sue's plants, making her sandwiches, helping her use the internet, and mailing letters for her were just as important as any other work I've done.

ONE MORNING, AT EXACTLY 8:00 A.M., I received a frantic phone call from our night-shift nurse. She told me that Ms. Sue had been unable to breathe overnight. The night nurse had gone over and tried to help her but, not surprisingly, Ms. Sue refused help and an ambulance. The nurse told me Ms. Sue was asking for me and wanted to know how quickly I could get to the home.

I got there within twenty-five minutes and was lucky I didn't get a speeding ticket as I raced down the highway. There I found Ms. Sue lying in her bed in her pajamas, which was alarming since she was always dressed and wearing her lipstick by 6:00 A.M. Something was really wrong. She had oxygen, but was still struggling to breathe. I felt panicky. By this point, Sue and I had spent several months together. I wasn't ready to lose her and hated seeing her suffer. After a few seconds of feeling overwhelmed by emotion, my training kicked in and I snapped into nurse mode. I administered her medications and increased her oxygen slightly until she was finally able to breathe normally and we were both able to relax, knowing that today was not *the* day.

I sat on the bed next to Sue, letting out a sigh of relief.

"I was really scared. I have never once doubted my faith, but I questioned it when I thought I was going to die," she said, looking directly at me.

I nodded and placed my hand over hers, repeating her own words from months ago back to her: "I think there are more people out there that have felt that way than would care to admit."

Soon, Ms. Sue's son arrived, and I showed him how to administer her medications to keep her pain-free. I left to go to my next patient's home, but told Ms. Sue that I would be on call 24/7. I could not stand the thought of her passing in pain. I was determined to be there with her in the end, in the way that I had been unable to for Mr. Carl, and I was sure to let everyone know to call me rather than the night nurse should the need arise.

Next, I called Steve, our chaplain. He was my grandparents' age and had been a chaplain for more than forty years. He was dependable, never missing a day of work that I know of, and enjoyed fishing on his days off. Although he didn't speak much of his personal life, occasionally we got to see a blurry photo of him holding up a fish that he had taken on his outdated flip phone. I never recognized him in the photos; his sunglasses, cut-off shorts, and flip-flops were a stark contrast from the tailored suits he wore to work. I had worked with him both in hospice and previously, at the nursing home. Steve truly cared about everyone he encountered and, over the years, both Chris and I had developed a relationship with him. While Steve was, of course, religious himself, he was there as a positive force for all of our patients, offering each person whatever they needed in the moment, whether they happened to be religious or not. Steve had gotten to know Ms. Sue during his weekly visits over the past several months. He told me that, although they read scripture and prayed together, he was never able to crack her tough exterior and truly get to know her.

"I think Ms. Sue is going to pass soon," I informed him.

"I'll go ahead and make the calls so we can get last rites for her," he assured me.

THE NEXT MORNING, I was standing at Ms. Sue's bedside with Steve. She was still struggling to breathe, but had improved from yesterday, thanks to her increased dose of morphine.

"He should be here any minute," Steve said.

As if on cue, an older man wearing long robes walked into Ms. Sue's room. I recognized him immediately, despite the fact that I hadn't seen him since that pivotal day in church with my mom, years before.

"Father Tom, good to see you, friend," Steve greeted him. "This is one of our nurses, Hadley, and this is Sue."

"Nice to meet you, Sue," Father Tom said as he knelt at her bedside. I felt shaky as I watched their interaction. Father Tom had no idea who I was, and yet he'd had such a huge impact on my life. As we bowed our heads in prayer, I listened to his voice, the voice I had heard in my head so many times over the years.

I was in a much different place now than when I was that pregnant nineteen-year-old in his congregation. I'd had my son, graduated nursing school, bought a home, and was supporting both of us by working full-time as a nurse. I had a boyfriend whom I wanted to marry one day. I wanted to tell Father Tom my story and explain how he changed my life, but the timing wasn't right. This moment was about Ms. Sue, and I tried my best to concentrate on his words as he prayed with her.

To end the ceremony, Father Tom had us all join hands and recite "Our Father." I knew it well, and I felt my heart swell as we all prayed in unison. It wasn't a religious feeling that moved me, just the sincere love I had for these three people in the room with me.

TWO NIGHTS LATER, the call came: Ms. Sue couldn't breathe. On the drive to her house, I wondered: How could I possibly be a good hospice nurse if I dreaded my patients' deaths? But that thought was quelled when I walked into her home and felt a sense of calm that I had never felt before. Ms. Sue was lying in her bed and struggling to breathe, but she was . . . smiling? *Must be the morphine,* I thought.

"How are you feeling?" I asked Sue while adjusting the oxygen under her nose.

"Excited. I can't wait to be with my husband. He's right beside you," she said.

I knew there was no one beside me, but by this point I was familiar enough with the phenomenon that I didn't question what Ms. Sue was seeing. I still felt a jolt run through me, though. In this case, it was less about the fact that she saw her husband, and more about the fact that this meant Ms. Sue's time was really coming to an end. I could sense that she was going to fall asleep soon, so I hurriedly asked her, "Are you scared?"

"No, he's here to get me. I finally get to be with him again," she said with a slight smile, her eyes closed.

I tried to smile in return. I was happy for Sue, but so sad to be losing her. Even though we'd been together for nine months, a few months longer than she was initially expected to live, I still wasn't ready. I drew up her medication, eyeballing the syringe to ensure the dosage was correct. As I knelt down to administer it, Sue opened her eyes and looked at me.

"He says we're going tonight," she rasped.

A tear rolled down my cheek. "Okay," I whispered. If I tried to say anything else, I knew I would lose it.

Sue was smiling. With her eyes still closed, she said, "Hey, I know that one day you'll have a long line of people waiting to greet you at the gates of Heaven, but they better get out of my way because I'll be the first one to hug you when you get there, okay?" After all these months of trying my best to offer comfort to Ms. Sue, to let her know I saw her, here she was comforting me.

I couldn't help it; I began sobbing. I attempted to wipe the snot and tears from my face, not wanting to put my feelings on Sue. After a few moments, I collected myself. I checked on her one last time before leaving, making sure that she was pain-free. She was sleeping, and she looked like an angel—perfectly at peace.

AS I GOT INTO bed that night, I feared the call would come at any moment.

I was surprised when I woke up to my alarm going off at 7:00 A.M. I checked my phone, panicking that I'd missed a call, but there was nothing. I poured myself some coffee and began getting ready for the day, checking every few minutes to make sure my ringer volume was set on high and that I hadn't missed a call. At 8:00 on the dot, I dialed Ms. Sue's son's number.

"Fred, it's Hadley. Is she doing okay?" I asked.

He paused briefly and then calmly told me, "She passed around three this morning. It was very peaceful. Your co-worker came and handled everything."

"I—I'm so sorry. I thought I told everyone that I would be on call so I could be there for her. There must have been a miscommunication. I'm so sorry," I stammered, shocked.

"Mom said not to call you when she died. She said that Dad told her that you couldn't handle it."

The tears fell freely as I let his words wash over me. He was right.

Although I had always known Ms. Sue's time was limited—just like all of my patients' time is—she had become a part of my life, a part of my routine. It was hard to imagine spending the 3:00 P.M. hour every Monday, Wednesday, and Friday any other way than with Ms. Sue, watering her plants, making her sandwiches, and doing anything else that might be helpful for her as she shared her stories with me.

A few days later, Steve came into my office holding a paper. "I think you'll want to see this," he said as he handed it to me.

It was Ms. Sue's obituary and, to my surprise, there was my name, along with a thank-you for taking care of her. I cried in disbelief as I read it. In the six years I've now been working in hospice, I've only been mentioned in three obituaries, and Ms. Sue's was the first. It felt so special to be included in this synopsis of Ms. Sue's long life, to be a part of how she would be remembered forever.

I will remember her forever too.

Sandra

I WAS SITTING IN MY CAR OUTSIDE THE HOUSE OF MY second patient of the day when Travis called. "Hey, Hadley! How's your day looking?"

"Swamped," I replied. I was already running behind and knew I would be skipping lunch.

"Well, I need you to do an admission near where you are right now."

"I have four more patients to see today. Can another nurse take the admission?" I protested, my voice climbing an octave.

"No," he replied curtly before hanging up the phone.

I could feel my stress levels rising as I looked up the phone numbers for the four patients remaining on my schedule. I prided myself on being consistent and reliable, which was another reason it irked me that I was being asked to move my schedule around. I called the first patient's son to tell him I had to move our appointment to later in the week. "Hadley, you can move us to any time you want as long as we get to see your smiling face," he replied in his thick Southern accent. I instantly relaxed.

Taking a second to breathe and focus, I opened my tablet and began reading about my new patient, Ms. Sandra. She was a fifty-year-old female with breast cancer who apparently needed immediate hospice admission. Guilt washed over me. How dare I get annoyed at a small inconvenience when someone's wife, mom, and best friend was dying? I skimmed over her medical history. She was diagnosed three months ago, and had tried chemotherapy and radiation, but the cancer had already spread to her bones, lungs, and liver. It was ravaging her body, which led the oncologist to recommend hospice. The "off the record" notes said that Sandra was in a terrible amount of pain and likely wouldn't survive another week. I plugged her address into my GPS and drove toward her house.

A few minutes later, I pulled into a sweeping driveway right off the beach. There was a bubbling fountain in the center of the driveway, and a Tesla sat outside the garage. (I wondered what they kept *inside* the garage, if that's what was on the outside.) Not surprisingly, the house was enormous. It was the type of house people dream of living in—absolute perfection.

I felt my confidence falter. Usually, the people who lived in homes like this didn't take well to listening to advice from a twenty-something nurse. I'd grown accustomed to hearing responses like "Well, I'll run it by my doctor friend before we make any decisions." I feared that would be particularly true in this case, with such a wealthy couple.

I put on my biggest customer-service smile, braced myself,

and knocked on the front door, where I was greeted by Sandra's husband, George, a tired-looking man in his fifties.
Without saying anything, he beckoned me in, then turned
around and walked back into the house. I hesitantly followed
him into the expansive foyer. Distracted by an enormous
chandelier the size of the Tesla in the driveway, it took me a
minute to realize that George was speaking to me, apologizing for being in a daze.

"It's absolutely fine," I reassured him. I looked around for
other family members or house staff, expecting to see someone cleaning the kitchen counters or mopping the floor, but
there was no one else.

The living room had floor-to-ceiling glass windows that
showcased a view of the water so spectacular that I felt like I
could reach out and touch it. Ms. Sandra was sitting on the
couch, gazing out the window. Not surprisingly, she was very
frail, though still well put together. I timidly introduced myself, explaining that I was from hospice. She turned to me and
I could see tears in her eyes.

"I am so glad you're here," she said. "I am in so much pain."

I started to worry. Getting medications at home is not as
simple as in the hospital, where you can call down to the
on-site pharmacy. I didn't want Ms. Sandra to suffer unneces-
sarily.

I asked what medications she had been taking for her pain
and she told me her husband had just given her Norco, a combination of acetaminophen (Tylenol) and hydrocodone (an
opioid). While it's an effective medication, it's often not
strong enough for cancer pain, especially when the cancer has

spread to the bones. My eyes widened as she told me she was on the lowest dose of Norco, and only taking it every six hours as prescribed.

Alarmed, I asked if I could call our physician. She nodded.

When I reached Dr. Kumar, I explained the situation to him.

"Jesus Christ," he said. "I will have a morphine prescription faxed to the pharmacy in the next two minutes."

I thanked him, feeling relieved. Then I turned to George and asked if there was someone else who could go to the pharmacy to pick up the prescription while he and I went through the admission process.

"It's just me here," he replied. "I don't think anyone else should care for my wife. This is my job." This was a first for me. Most wealthy people have an arsenal of paid people at their disposal.

I called the closest pharmacy and the robotic prerecorded voice told me its hours and locations, then proceeded to run me through an advertisement for flu shot specials. I tried in vain to press zero to reach a human. The minute-long recording felt like an hour as I watched the tears roll down Ms. Sandra's face.

Finally, a pharmacy tech answered. "I need a pharmacist please," I said urgently. "My doctor is faxing over a prescription and I need it filled ASAP for a hospice patient." I heard a click. My mouth fell open in shock, thinking the tech had hung up on me. Thankfully, I soon heard another voice—the pharmacist. *Thank goodness.* I explained the situation and he told me to give him fifteen minutes. I thanked him and hung up, feeling grateful. Pharmacists don't have to go out of their way for hospice workers, but we always appreciate it when they do.

As soon as George left for the pharmacy, I called Dr. Kumar and asked him what we could do to give Ms. Sandra some relief while we waited for her husband to return. He instructed me to give her an extra Norco. While we waited for it to kick in, I rubbed Sandra's back and spoke to her in a calm voice, but she was still whimpering from the pain. I picked up the remote on the coffee table and pressed play. The soothing voice of Norah Jones soon filled the room. I continued rubbing her back as we silently watched the waves outside the window crash into the shore. It seemed to help some, but not much. When her husband came home with the bag from the pharmacy in hand, I asked Ms. Sandra if she was still in pain. She nodded through her tears, and I gave her the smallest dose of morphine to make sure she didn't have an adverse reaction to the medication.

An hour after I had arrived, Ms. Sandra was finally relaxed, pain-free, and sleeping soundly. I could see the weight lift from her husband's shoulders. "Thank you," he said quietly to me. "I haven't seen her relax in months. It was killing me." He turned his face away quickly, but I saw him grimace at his poor choice of words. I nodded in understanding.

"The next dose can be given in an hour and a half. Let's write out a schedule along with some other things, so you aren't trying to remember too much."

"Thanks. That sounds great. I'm really lost and tired."

I walked over to my nursing bag and pulled out my notebook and pen. "She received morphine thirty minutes ago. It's two o'clock now, and the doctor said she can have it every two hours as needed." George nodded. "Now," I said, "can I explain how we determine pain in case she can't tell you?"

"Why wouldn't she be able to tell me?" he asked.

I paused. This poor man had already had a lot thrown at him. Maybe it was best to not overwhelm him today. Then I remembered the oncologist's note: *will not survive another week*. "Sometimes at the end of life, people lose their ability to communicate," I said as gently as possible. "Usually, it looks like they're just sleeping all the time."

George's eyes widened as he looked at his sleeping wife.

"That's not what's happening right now," I quickly assured him. George relaxed somewhat but I could tell he was still tense. "It's been a lot today. How about I come by tomorrow?" I suggested.

"That would be wonderful. Thank you, Hadley."

I WALKED OUT TO my car and checked my text messages. I had a message from Chris asking me to call him. My heart rate sped up. He never sent texts like that when I was working.

The phone rang twice before he picked up. "Hey, it's my mom. We're in the emergency room." A sense of dread immediately set in. Before Chris and I had met, his mom, Babette, had been diagnosed with glioblastoma, an aggressive form of brain cancer. She was just fifty-three at the time, and was originally given just a few months to live. Yet she was still here almost two years later. We knew we were on borrowed time, and the days when she had scans were always a cause for either celebration or devastation, but at this point she seemed to be stable. On the last MRI, the tumors hadn't grown.

On some days, it was easy to forget Babette was sick at all. A former nurse herself, she was a spitfire, and she never appeared ill. In fact, I was always amazed by how healthy she looked, based on the hospice patients I worked with who also suffered from brain cancer and definitely didn't look healthy. Despite these appearances, Babette's impending death loomed over us like a rain cloud; we were unsure when it would begin to rain, but knew that we'd soon be drenched if we didn't find shelter. Except there was no shelter, no place to escape. So we were just standing there waiting for the rain, waiting for phone calls like this.

I WAS INTIMIDATED WHEN I first met Chris's parents, just a few weeks after we started dating. We had met another couple while playing beach volleyball on one of our first dates, and they'd invited us to join them for a weekend in New Orleans. It was early on in our relationship, but we decided to go for it—it sounded like fun, and my mom was willing to watch Brody. When Chris told his parents that we were going away together, they insisted on meeting me first.

On top of all the usual jitters that come from meeting a new boyfriend's family, I was concerned that Chris's parents wouldn't like the fact that I was a single mom. I imagined that wasn't exactly what a mother dreamed about for her single doctor son. It also made me nervous that Babette had been a nurse herself. She had started out as a school nurse, rising through the ranks until she was president of the Georgia Association of School Nurses, which served all the school nurses in the entire state of Georgia. She'd had to step down from that role shortly after her diagnosis, and I knew it devastated her.

On the night we met his parents for dinner, I nervously adjusted the skirt of my dress as Chris pulled his car into the parking lot outside the waterfront restaurant. "They're going to love you," Chris said, sensing my nerves.

I smiled and nodded, not quite sure if that was true, before exiting the car and walking into the restaurant on his arm.

As we approached the table, I saw a man in a nice button-down shirt, his gray hair slicked back, and a very petite woman with blond hair sitting next to him. There were two open seats across from them. Chris's dad, Tom, saw us first and motioned to Babette that we had arrived. Chris introduced me as his parents stood up to greet us.

"Hi." I smiled, hoping they couldn't tell how awkward I felt. If they did, there was no indication. Tom and Babette took turns hugging both Chris and me, and almost instantly I felt more comfortable.

After we sat down, Babette turned to me. "I heard you're a nurse," she said.

"I am," I replied, sipping my water and nodding.

"Tell me about your schooling."

I looked at Chris, a little shocked at how forward Babette was, but he was occupied talking to his dad. "Well, I became a registered nurse about a year ago," I started.

"Will you always work as a nurse? I heard you have a baby."

"Yes, I plan on it," I said.

"I stayed home when the kids were young," Babette shared.

"It's important. Careers will always be there." That must have gotten Chris's attention because he quickly interrupted to bring Babette and me into the conversation he and Tom were having about New Orleans.

When we left dinner later that evening, Babette made sure to tell Chris how much she loved him and how proud she was of him. I left feeling like Chris had amazing parents, but wasn't so sure that Babette liked that I already had a child. Plus, they were clearly such a close-knit family that it was hard to imagine how Brody and I might fit in. I was sure that Chris would tell me my fears were nonsense if I brought them up, but being a young single mom had made me hyperaware of others' judgments—and my concerns often turned out to be well-founded.

Although we had only been together for a short time, Chris was . . . different, and I already knew that I wanted to marry him. But in moments like this, I couldn't help but wonder if that white-picket-fence life I dreamed of for Brody and me was outside of our reach.

IN THE YEAR SINCE that first meeting, as both Brody and I had grown in our relationship with Chris, we had grown closer to Babette and Tom, as well. As I drove to the hospital, I thought about how I wasn't ready to lose her.

I was momentarily blinded by the bright overhead lights as I stepped into the emergency room lobby. I trained to become a nurse at this very hospital, and spent another year as a paid intern in this exact emergency room. As I walked back through the emergency room halls looking for Chris and his family, I saw a group huddled at the nurses' station talking. I knew almost all of them.

I couldn't help but overhear as a nurse with her back turned toward me spoke. "What do they expect us to do? She has cancer. We can't cure her. This is a waste of my time." As I walked up, the nurse turned around. I stopped in my tracks: It was Theresa, the nurse who had trained me—someone I looked up to, someone I idolized and wanted to emulate. There was no doubt in my mind it was Babette she was speaking about.

Theresa and I made eye contact, but neither of us said a word. I couldn't pretend like I hadn't always known who Theresa was. Of course I did; I'd seen her interact with patients plenty of times before. But, suddenly, I vividly understood how wrong I'd been. Each of those patients was someone else's Babette, someone else's loved one. It was a sickening realization. And as I looked at the nurses gathered around the station who hadn't participated, but also hadn't admonished Theresa, I couldn't help but think how I'd done the same when I was with her, remaining silent and compliant, even in those moments when I disagreed with how she treated a patient or their loved one.

I turned away when I heard Chris's voice, calling me from where he stood in the doorway of room four. Before joining him, I made eye contact with Theresa one more time. Throughout this entire exchange, we never spoke a word to each other.

Inside of the room, Babette smiled at me from the hospital bed, but I could tell she was weak. Tom sat in a chair at her bedside, a stoic but stabilizing force. He held Babette's hand and kept an eye on the hospital monitor as it began to take her blood pressure again.

"What do you think is wrong?" I asked Babette.

"I think it's the flu or an infection of some sort," she replied. "I tried to get in to see my regular doctor, but he told me to come here. I don't want to be in the ER, but he said I need treatment before I can continue my chemotherapy."

I nodded and stepped out of the way as Theresa walked in and began hitting buttons on the monitor, pulling up Babette's latest readings.

"Looks good," Theresa said, as she began twisting a syringe with clear liquid in it onto Babette's IV access.

Babette pulled her hand back slightly. "Wait, what are you giving me?" she asked.

"I don't have to give it to you," Theresa said as she unscrewed the medication.

"I'm not refusing it, I just want to know what it is," Babette clarified.

"A medicine your doctor ordered. Want to take it up with him?"

When I trained under Theresa, I admired her "no BS" nursing, as she called it. Now, I realized that it was just rudeness. Babette looked like she was ready to fight Theresa, but Tom, always the peacekeeper, stepped in.

"If we could just get the name of the medicine, I think that's all we need. We appreciate you," he said to Theresa.

THE NEXT MORNING, I called the report line to see if any of my patients had called the night before. "Ms. Betty fell. I went out and checked her out. She had a skin tear to her right arm. Check on her again today, please, and replace the bandage tomorrow. Mr. Robert called an hour ago to ask where you were. I reminded him that it was seven in the morning and that you would call him around nine. That was it." I was surprised there was no call from Ms. Sandra.

After hanging up with my co-worker, I called Ms. Sandra's husband.

"Hey, Hadley!" George answered, sounding very different from the day before.

"How was y'all's night?" I asked.

"Great! We got to sleep. I woke Sandra up twice to give her medications but otherwise we slept great. We're outside eating breakfast now. She asked for coffee—she hasn't asked for coffee in months!" He was jubilant. I smiled to myself as I was reminded of the power of pain control.

"Can I come see y'all this morning?" I asked.

"We can't wait to see you!"

One hour later, I was greeted at the massive front door by a completely different man than the one I'd met yesterday. George no longer looked tired, and he was dressed in a suit with a cup of coffee in his hands.

Ms. Sandra was sitting on the couch, smiling, and I instantly smiled too. I went through my usual routine of checking vital signs and assessing all body systems as her husband finished up what sounded like a business phone call.

"Working today?" I asked George.

"It never ends!" he exclaimed. I turned to Ms. Sandra and asked, "What about you? Did you work?"

"Oh, honey," she replied, "I was a professional housewife. I got the best of both worlds. Love *and* money." Now that she was out of pain, Sandra oozed warmth and good humor. I laughed with her and finished up my charting before leaving, promising I would be back in a few days.

The weeks came and went without incident as Sandra proceeded to exceed her doctor's initial one-week diagnosis. I was reminded again how critical pain management is. Yes, Sandra still had cancer and she was terminal, but she was *living* now. She was happy. Our routine visits included lots of laughs as I learned more about my remarkable patient. It turns out "professional housewife" was a self-effacing title; Ms. Sandra had actually run multiple nonprofit organizations in the area that benefited foster children.

After a couple of months like this, Ms. Sandra slowly declined, though she was able to keep her pain at bay in the process. She ultimately lost the ability to walk, but George was by her side the entire time, and even learned how to transfer her safely to a wheelchair with my direction. The smile never left Ms. Sandra's face as her husband lovingly cared for her. And, true to his word, he never allowed another person to touch her. Extended family came and went, each person kinder than the one before and grateful that hospice had given Sandra back her quality of life, even if just for the moment.

Despite their power and prestige, Sandra and George trusted me and allowed me to make the decisions that would help them. In my time with them, I felt empowered to make suggestions and continued to build my confidence as a nurse. And they were also a good reminder that, no matter what our different circumstances might be, death is a part of life for each and every one of us—there is no white picket fence we can build that's strong enough to waylay the natural course of things. When the time comes, we all want the same things: care, comfort, and connection.

ONE DAY ABOUT THREE months after admitting Ms. Sandra to hospice, I was sitting in my office eating lunch when my phone rang. I was slightly surprised to see it was Ms. Sandra's home number; she and George had never once called, and I had just left their house on a routine visit a couple of hours before.

"Hadley," George said when I answered the phone, "something is different."

I felt a lump in my throat as I put down my sandwich and grabbed my car keys. As I drove, I told myself as I had before that I couldn't get so emotionally attached to patients; it's how hospice nurses burn out and end up quitting. I slammed on my brakes as a tourist walked out in front of my car, flipping me the bird and yelling at me. *It must be nice to be able to go to the beach right now,* I thought.

I pulled into the now-familiar driveway. As I got out of the car, I shielded my eyes from the bright sun, taking a second to soak in the chirping birds and lovely light breeze. I am continually amazed at how life just continues on as usual, despite the tragedy that exists all around us.

George opened the door before I could knock and ushered me inside. Ms. Sandra was lying on the hospital bed, facing the windows that looked out to the beautiful view of the water. I knew something was different, too—the silence in the house was palpable. Earlier this morning, Ms. Sandra had been weak, but talking. Now she was not. I reached for her hand. It was ice-cold. I worried that she might have already passed, but then I heard her take a ragged breath. She was actively passing, I realized, and I informed George, using gentler words. I gave her medications to ensure her comfort, then sat down opposite him.

"How much longer?" he asked.

"At this point, I would say about seventy-two hours or less."

George sighed heavily and rubbed his face, then said, "Okay. Our only daughter is on her way from Chicago. She should be here within the hour."

"I'm going to stay for now to monitor Ms. Sandra, if that is okay with you."

"I would prefer that. Any suggestions for what to do now?"

"We could play some of that soft music she likes," I suggested.

George nodded and left the room. He returned a minute later with a small portable radio and an essential oil diffuser in hand. "She loves this thing."

"Perfect," I said, giving him an encouraging smile.

We plugged in the diffuser and played some Norah Jones in the background. A scent that evoked the sea wafted through the air as George and I sat across from each other and he told me stories about Ms. Sandra as a mother. He talked about how she'd devoted her life to their daughter, how they were "two peas in a pod," how they spoke every day, even as adults. My heart ached for their daughter, who was about to walk into one of the most difficult days of her life.

When George's daughter called to let him know that she was in the rental car leaving the airport, I noticed he didn't tell her that her mother's passing was imminent. As if reading my mind, he told me, "I don't want to tell her on the phone and risk a car accident." I nodded, understanding. George continued telling me stories while holding his wife's hand. He had tears in his eyes, but he was also smiling as he reminisced about their happy times.

In the middle of a sentence, the air in the room suddenly grew heavier. George stopped talking and we both turned to look at Sandra. After a moment of silence, he asked, "What do I do?".

Without hesitating like I normally did when making big decisions, I confidently told him, "Keep holding her hand and talking." I held Ms. Sandra's other hand and silently prayed that her daughter would arrive quickly.

As George was telling Sandra how much he loved her, I heard the front door open. Relief washed over me.

"Hey, Mom and Dad!" a voice rang out from the foyer. "I'm going to put my bags in the guest room. Be there in a minute."

Still holding Ms. Sandra's hand, I heard myself speak. "Come here right now!" I yelled to their daughter, surprised by my own assertiveness.

A moment later, I moved from Ms. Sandra's bedside so her daughter could hold her mother's hand. Shocked at what she saw, she cried out, and kissed her mother's forehead, telling her how much she loved her.

At that exact same moment, I watched as Ms. Sandra, beloved mother and wife, took her final breath.

TO THIS DAY, I still think about how miraculous it was that Ms. Sandra's daughter made it to her side, just as her mother took her last breath. I think about Sandra and how she was a mom to the end, holding on for as long as she could so that she could hold her child's hand one last time. There's no doubt in my mind that the timing of her daughter's arrival and Sandra's departure was not a coincidence.

One of the more stunning and beautiful things I've witnessed as a hospice nurse is the way in which people choose their time of death. So many of us can't choose when we go to *sleep* at night, and yet we seem to have some control over when we die. I've had some patients intent on dying alone, stealing away in the matter of seconds they're left to themselves while a loved one goes to the bathroom, and others, like Sandra, who hang on until the moment when a loved one reaches their side.

I've seen this enough times that I shouldn't be surprised at this point, but it never ceases to amaze and fascinate me.

Elizabeth

CHRISTMAS MUSIC WAS PLAYING ON THE RADIO AS I drove up to Elizabeth's home on a gloomy winter's day. She lived in a quiet cul-de-sac a few miles from the beach, a middle-class neighborhood that would be considered upper-class anywhere else.

Elizabeth's sister, who introduced herself as Julia and appeared to be in her forties, answered the door and beckoned me in. The house behind her was silent, except for the sound of the dishwasher lightly buzzing in the background.

"Are you the nurse's aide?" she asked once I'd stepped into the house.

"I'm the nurse," I said, making every effort to keep my tone calm and confident. Although I was twenty-five years old and had been a nurse for a year and a half, many patients told me I didn't even look eighteen. I was even more self-conscious about my young age because I was so different from all of the other nurses I worked with, most of whom came to hospice as a second career.

Julia smiled wryly. "Well, I'd say we're happy to see you, but it kind of feels like you're the angel of death."

I nodded in understanding. "Do you live here with her?" I asked.

"Nope. I have two kids and a husband to tend to, but I do live right down the street and I come here often. I'm a stay-at-home mom. Elizabeth doesn't talk to anyone else in the family." Julia paused for a moment before continuing, "No one expected this, though. We all thought Dad would be the next to go, with his heart and all. I don't know how this happened . . ." She trailed off, looking at the floor.

I nodded. "I promise I'll take good care of her."

She sighed heavily and replied, "It's life, I guess." Julia wiped her nose and motioned down the hallway to our left. "She's in there. You can go ahead."

I nodded and headed in the direction Julia indicated. All I knew about Elizabeth was what I had read in her chart: *Forty years old. Lung cancer. History of surgery and chemotherapy with no success. Nonsmoker. No family history of lung cancer. Unknown cause.* I couldn't imagine being given such a devastating diagnosis with no explanation as to why. I prepared myself for an angry patient. I had learned early on that many cancer patients take out their anger on the hospice nurses. I tried not to take it personally when that happened, but that was harder to do some days than others.

As I entered the room, the first thing I noticed was a candle burning on Elizabeth's nightstand and the smell of lemon mixed with linen. It struck me as a clean, hopeful scent. Next, I noticed a smiling face. "Aren't you the cutest little thing?" I heard Elizabeth say.

A genuine smile crept across my face, and I felt a tiny bit of relief sweep through me.

Elizabeth was a beautiful woman who looked much younger than forty. She had blond hair, blue eyes, and the skin of a porcelain doll. She was thin, but had very toned arms, which were visible thanks to the sleeveless purple tank top she was wearing.

"I need to take your vital signs, if that's okay," I said, momentarily intimidated by her beauty.

"Of course, honeybunch!" Elizabeth replied sweetly. It was clear that she could tell I was a little nervous and was trying to make me feel as comfortable as possible.

As I wrapped the blood pressure cuff around her arm, I asked if she worked out a lot.

She sighed and smiled. "Well, I used to teach yoga. Not anymore, though."

I nodded and felt myself flush. I should have known better than to have asked that. Of course she couldn't work out anymore. "125/70," I reported, as I entered the numbers into my tablet.

"You must work out too," Elizabeth said.

"I do."

As I finished up the rest of my assessment, Elizabeth asked when she would see me next.

"Well, you can call this number at any time and a nurse is always available to come see you. I can plan to come back later this week, if that works for you?"

"Sounds wonderful, Hadley."

———

JULIA WALKED ME OUT and watched me back down the driveway, as if she was making sure I didn't hit the mailbox on my way out. While she had been perfectly nice on the surface, Julia seemed to lack her sister's warmth. It felt like she was watching me, judging, wondering if I was up to the job.

As I drove to my next patient, I replayed my visit with Elizabeth. I cringed as I remembered asking her about working out. Just that morning, I had gotten out of bed and looked in the bathroom mirror, mentally picking apart my appearance. I stepped onto the cold scale and waited for the results. I watched the zero *blink, blink, blink* and then the number 115 appear on the small screen. I sighed and scolded myself for splitting a slice of pie with Chris the night before. As I pulled on my black tennis shoes and tied my hair up into a messy bun, I worried that he would leave me if I didn't stay as skinny as I was when we first met. I had to stay at or below 112 pounds, I reminded myself.

I WAS FOURTEEN YEARS OLD when my eating disorder kicked in. I was sitting on a barstool at our kitchen counter after school, doing my English homework. The smell of garlic was heavy in the air and *Jeopardy!* played on the television behind me in the living room.

"Oh, I know this one! It's China!" my mom exclaimed, waving a wooden spatula in the air. Looking satisfied, she stirred the bubbling liquid on the stovetop. We laughed when Alex Trebek said, "The correct answer is Japan."

"You definitely knew that one, Mom," I teased her.

I grabbed another chip from the bag next to me and happily bit into it. My mom took another swig of her red wine and began reciting her cooking tips, once again expressing her hope that I would someday cook for my own family. She talked with her hands and her eyes lit up whenever she discussed cooking.

We heard the front door open and we both looked in that direction. I grabbed another chip from the bag as my dad quickly walked past me and into the kitchen without acknowledging me.

I breathed a sigh of relief. My dad was very strict and also unpredictable, which meant that I was always on guard. On good days, he might play the guitar on the porch and grill a delicious dinner for the family, all while talking about how my brothers and I were the best kids ever. And then, on bad days, so much as a pillow out of place on my bed could be enough to warrant him telling me that I would never find a husband since no one would ever love or want to marry a messy girl like me.

"What's wrong?" my mom asked meekly. She was hunching her shoulders, as if to make herself smaller.

"I've been thinking," he said as he paced in the kitchen. Back and forth he walked, running his hands through his hair. I knew something bad was coming. I stayed as still as possible, hoping that the words wouldn't be flung in my direction. "I just never thought I would marry someone who was fat," he said, spitting the words at her.

My eyes widened as I watched my mom stirring the pot on the stovetop. Although her back was to me, I could tell she was trying her best to hide the fact that she was crying.

My dad sighed heavily when he realized she wasn't going to respond, and walked out the front door once again.

In many ways, this was a fairly typical day in my childhood—at the time, it felt normal to me, even though I now understand it was not normal behavior at all. But on this particular day, something landed a bit different. Suddenly, I was no longer hungry. Not for the chips and not for dinner. I stared at my mom's back and waist and mentally compared them to mine. She looked just like me, so I came to the conclusion that my dad must think that I was fat too.

Before that day, I hadn't been aware of my body at all. Looking back, I can see that I was very slim, but I didn't feel like that at the time. I began to notice when my dad asked if I *really* needed to eat a second helping at dinnertime. I grew hyperaware of my body and was diligent about making sure that I stayed a certain size, no matter what. I knew that my dad was aware of what size I was, because he took me clothes shopping when I got all A's and B's on my report card, and commented on those trips that he loved that I was a size zero.

Although these memories stand out in my mind, it would be wrong to blame these issues on one person, who I'm sure had his own reasoning for how he chose to parent. My eating disorder was exacerbated by society as well—teen magazines that advertised "Five Ways to Lose Five Pounds by the Holidays" were extremely commonplace during those years. I internalized the conversations of adults who talked about their own weight, and the latest fad diet they were on as well.

During my high school years, I saw the number on the scale as I saw my grades: a direct reflection of my worth. High grades and a low number on the scale were a reason to celebrate, and the opposite results meant that I had to work overtime for others to love and accept me.

———

MY OBSESSION WITH MY weight continued throughout college and nursing school, and even into the earlier days of my career. My weight-control method of choice was a combination of bingeing and purging and avoiding food altogether. When I was pregnant with Brody, I threw up every day due to hyperemesis gravidarum. I was convinced that it was karma for all the times I had forced myself to vomit, though my mom assured me it was not (and I now understand that, too).

During nursing school, I was caught in a constant cycle of worrying about bills, caring for a baby, and trying to keep my grades up so I wouldn't lose my scholarships. The only thing I felt like I had control over was my weight.

In reality, I was not in control of anything. I was good at hiding what I was doing, though. The only person who seemed to notice was my teacher, Professor Lopez, likely because she was a psych nurse.

"Have you eaten?" she sometimes asked me at clinicals, the twelve-hour days we spent learning in the hospital.

"I'm busy today," I responded, shrugging.

"I'm headed down to the cafeteria. What do you want? It's on me," Ms. Lopez responded with a warm smile. "You can't learn anything on an empty stomach."

ONE DAY IN CLASS, Ms. Lopez motioned for me to come up to her desk. We were all at our computers completing a practice test, and the only sound in the room was the air conditioner humming.

"How are you feeling about the test on Monday?" she asked when I approached her.

"I'll be okay," I replied.

"Your practice scores say differently. You know you have to get at least a seventy-four on this test to stay in the program. What's going on?"

I hesitated. Other than my friend Summer, I was the youngest in the class and the only single mom. Most of my classmates were my parents' age.

"My son isn't sleeping," I confessed. "He's teething and needs me to hold him all the time. I used to be able to give him toys and read my textbook aloud to him, but it's not working anymore. I can't get any studying done."

Ms. Lopez nodded and rubbed her chin in thought. "Meet me at my office bright and early Saturday morning. Bring your son and your textbooks."

I nodded in agreement, unsure what the plan was.

WHEN I SHOWED UP on Saturday with my fussy son in one hand and my textbook in the other, Ms. Lopez greeted me with her big smile and took Brody into her arms.

"Someone won't let Mommy study, huh?" she said in a soothing voice. "Mommy is going to be right here, and you and I are going to play quietly. If Mommy doesn't understand something, I'm going to help her."

A wave of relief washed over me. Like a flash, I began unpacking my textbooks, wanting to make the most of this opportunity.

Professor Lopez spent her entire Saturday with Brody and

me. I walked out of her office feeling much more prepared for my test on Monday than I had when I entered. I even had a few more hours to study when I got home, since Brody had fallen asleep in his car seat. She had worn him out.

On Monday morning, I dropped Brody off at daycare and confidently walked in to take my test. We usually had to wait a few hours for our grades to be updated online, but as I walked out of the computer lab and past Professor Lopez's office, she made a beeline for me.

"You did it, Mama!" she said, hugging me. "Eighty-six percent. I'm so proud of you."

I hugged her back through tears of relief and gratitude.

Professor Lopez was one of those people who really saw me, who believed in my worth, and who made a difference. It's amazing how even those people who are in our life for just a short time can make a lasting impact.

A FEW DAYS AFTER our first visit, I was at Elizabeth's bedside again. It was Christmas Eve, and I was trying to fit in all of my patients so that I could rejoin Brody at Chris's parents' house. We'd just finished up a birthday lunch with balloons, cake, and presents, and now I was off to visit all of the patients who needed me before I could celebrate Christmas. One of the hierarchical rules in the nursing world is that newer nurses always work the holidays. My first year in nursing, I had naively requested Christmas Eve off to celebrate Brody's birthday, only to be told that I should have become a teacher if I expected to have any holidays off. Whenever I felt resentful about working on Christmas Eve, I reminded myself of the nurses who had been away from their family to take care of Brody and me on the night I gave birth. It made those holidays slightly more bearable.

This time Elizabeth had a little white dog sleeping happily next to her in bed while I completed her assessment. I was glad that at least she wasn't completely alone on Christmas.

"Any pain?" I asked.

"None at all," she said. "I'm fortunate in that way."

"How about any nausea or vomiting?" I momentarily thought about my own vomiting that morning, albeit for a completely different reason.

"None. Just lots of weakness," she said. I filled in the appropriate boxes and continued my assessment. Elizabeth politely answered all of my questions.

As I paused and contemplated what to type next, Elizabeth said, "Hey, can I get something off my chest?"

I immediately put away my tablet, placing it in my bag at my feet to give her my full attention. "Yes, of course."

"I have had a lot of time to just sit here and think. There's not much else to do."

I nodded and leaned forward, wanting her to feel encouraged to continue.

"I think I wasted a lot of my life on the treadmill."

This was not where I was expecting this conversation to go, but I was intrigued.

"I keep thinking about all the times when I was invited to the beach with my friends and didn't go because of the way my stomach looked. All the birthday dinners I skipped because I made all my own meals so I could obsessively count calories. I even skipped out on having friends over on my birthday because I didn't want to have to eat cake."

I realized I wasn't breathing. "That definitely resonates with me," I told her, while looking at the floor, ashamed that it must have been obvious.

Elizabeth looked me dead in the eyes and said, "I felt like I had to tell you this because I see myself in you. I never anticipated dying at forty. I always thought I would have more time. I wish I would have spent more time with my loved ones. I wish I'd just eaten the damn cake."

"That's good advice," I said softly. "Eat the cake."

"Eat the cake," she repeated, lying back in her bed.

I finished the rest of my charting in silence and said my goodbyes to Elizabeth, promising to see her again on Monday.

I MULLED OVER HER words as I drove to Chris's parents' house. The only time people had ever commented on my weight was to tell me how good I looked. This was usually after I had lost a few pounds, or when I "bounced back" so quickly after Brody's birth because I'd been so nauseous throughout my pregnancy and then immediately started running around after he arrived, trying to do it all and set up a stable situation for us. The validation always felt great. No one ever asked why I skipped dinners with friends or never ate sweets, but much like Professor Lopez had known something wasn't quite right, Elizabeth seemed to as well. It was almost like she could see right through me.

As I pulled into the parking lot of Babette and Tom's condo, I freshened up my lipstick in the rearview mirror and tried to pep myself up. Somehow, Babette was always in a positive mood despite her diagnosis, even when her scans didn't come in looking great, as they had this week. I felt it was necessary to match her positivity, even though I was dead tired both mentally and physically.

I could smell dinner cooking as soon as I opened the front door to Babette and Tom's home. It was filled with relatives who'd come from out of town to celebrate, brimming with festivity. As soon as I entered, I was greeted by the sight of Brody sitting on a big green armchair with Babette and all of her grandchildren reading *The Night Before Christmas,* a family tradition. Chris got off the couch to give me a hug and kiss as I watched, feeling like my heart was going to burst. Brody and I were part of something bigger—we were part of a family.

After they had finished the story, Babette called out, "All right, everyone! Time for ornaments!" I grabbed my wineglass and found a spot on the couch as Babette pulled out the family's ornaments. When she got to one that read BEST NURSE EVER, she said, "Hadley, do you want to do the honors?" Smiling, I stood up and took the ornament, carefully placing it on an empty tree limb. "Only the best men choose nurses, huh, honey?" Babette said, winking at Tom.

My heart hurt for her momentarily, knowing how fleeting it all was. It hurt for Chris, who was aware that this was almost certainly the last Christmas he would ever spend with his mother. And it hurt for me, knowing that this strong, spitfire of a woman whom I'd grown to love—who had clearly accepted me and my son into her family—wouldn't be a part of my family's future.

We all ate dinner, some family members sitting at the small wooden table and others dispersed throughout the living room. When we were finishing up, Babette called out, "Okay, who wants cheesecake?"

Chris politely declined and turned toward me for my answer. It would have been easy to say no after he had declined (as I normally would have), but cheesecake sounded delicious and Elizabeth's words were still ringing in my ears. Tonight I was going to eat the cake.

"I would love some," I said.

Chris raised his eyebrows in surprise. "Changed my mind. I'll have some too, Mom."

I enjoyed every bite of that cheesecake while I soaked in this moment of family, of belonging, of recognizing that Brody and I were exactly where I had always wished we would be.

On the drive home, I didn't think about the food digesting in my stomach like I normally would have. Instead, I smiled and gazed out at the Christmas lights twinkling as Chris talked about the Christmas morning his family got their dog, Holly. I silently thanked Elizabeth, just as I've thanked her a million times since then, because although I have had moments of weakness regarding my eating disorder, I have never relapsed since that night.

When we got home, Chris and I quietly carried a sleeping Brody in from the car and tucked him in bed. Then our work began, as we set to building the ginormous fire station Santa was bringing Brody that year. Hours passed as Chris attached tiny parts for what seemed like an eternity. I looked at the clock and saw it was 3:00 A.M. "I think that's good enough," I told him, surveying our work. "He won't even notice those parts are missing."

Chris didn't look up from tightening the world's tiniest screw with the world's tiniest screwdriver. "Santa doesn't do good enough. Santa only does perfect," he muttered.

AFTER LESS THAN AN hour of sleep, I woke up before the sun on Christmas morning and made sure all of the presents were in their proper place. I couldn't wait to see the excitement on Brody's face when he saw what Santa had brought for him. This was the first year that I could afford everything he wanted. In years past, I had tried to put aside ten to fifteen dollars per month for Christmas so that he could have at least one gift from Santa. He would open his one present and curl up next to me, his little body so warm, as I scrolled through Facebook, envious of all the other "normal" families whose large living rooms were filled with toys for their children. I vowed to be able to do that one day for Brody—and finally, I had.

Just then, Brody's bedroom door opened and I heard the sound of his little feet running, powered by Christmas morning excitement. As soon as he entered the living room his face lit up with joy. Chris joined us and we all sat around opening presents, then dove into a steaming stack of pancakes.

As we were eating, my phone rang. I was on call today and had a few patients scheduled, but I wasn't supposed to start for at least thirty more minutes. Will, our eleventh-hour volunteer and a saint in my eyes, was on the other end of the line.

His job was to sit with patients who had no one else so they wouldn't die alone. Usually, that meant staying overnight with them. "Merry Christmas!" he said.

"Merry Christmas," I replied. "I haven't gotten the report yet. Did you have an eleventh hour? On Christmas Eve?"

"Yes. Ms. Elizabeth."

I stopped mid-bite. Hers was the absolute last name I was expecting Will to say. She had been fine other than some weakness the day before.

"I'm so sorry, Will. I'm shocked. Do you need me to come there so you can go see your family for Christmas?"

"No—I'm fine. Her sister wants an update, but I don't know what to tell her. Travis said to call you because she's on your schedule today."

"I can leave here in just a few minutes," I promised.

I PULLED UP AT Elizabeth's house to the sight of her Christmas lights merrily lighting up the palm trees that framed it. It was the perfect Florida Christmas scene. If anyone drove by, it would probably conjure up images of a joyful Christmas morning inside the house. Little would they know that someone inside was spending their last moments on Earth.

I walked in without knocking, hoping to provide the sense of a familiar presence to Elizabeth. When I walked into her room, Will was sitting in the chair at her bedside. I smiled and thanked him profusely for being there. He said goodbye to Elizabeth with a wave and I began assessing her so that I could provide Julia with an update. Her face was makeup-free and pale, and her blond hair was disheveled. Her fingers were light blue and cold to the touch. I pulled the sheet up to just below her chest, and took out my stethoscope to listen to her heart and lungs. Her heart rate was sporadic, and she was alternating between fast and slow breaths. Her lungs sounded like Rice Krispies, an indicator that fluid had built up in them.

I sanitized my hands and pulled out my phone to call Julia. When she answered, I could hear her family enjoying Christmas morning in the background. I told her that it probably wouldn't be much longer and she should come over now. She said she would be over as soon as she could, but it was important for her kids not to have a Christmas morning without their mom there. "One day when you have kids you'll understand, dear," she explained.

When I hung up I could feel that something wasn't right in the room. I started talking to Elizabeth even though I knew she wouldn't respond. As I racked my brain to figure out how to make the atmosphere more "Elizabeth," I heard the front door open. *Thank goodness,* I thought, *Julia changed her mind.*

"Oh, Ms. Elizabeth!" Confused, I turned to find not Julia, but Deja, one of our nursing aides. As always, her makeup was done and her hair hung down her back in braids. I was glad to see her. Like me, Deja was young, but she also had a calm, motherly sort of energy about her—I felt safe and comfortable every time I was around her, as did patients. There was no doubt she would make a wonderful nurse, and I always encouraged her to go to nursing school. Deja was also a single mom, and we'd bonded over our similar situations. "Merry Christmas!" she said, pulling me into a hug. "I heard and came right away. I knew you'd be here too."

"You didn't have to leave your son on Christmas morning. You could have waited," I told her.

"I can't let you be the only one gettin' all that praise in the office," Deja replied with a chuckle. "Now, let's get our friend lookin' more like herself."

Deja began rummaging through Elizabeth's nightstand and pulled out a candle. As the room filled with a clean, light lemon scent, it started to feel much more like the peaceful environment I had come to know. I picked up the remote and flicked through the channels until I found the instrumental music station that Elizabeth loved.

"Ms. Elizabeth, Hadley and I are going to get you cleaned up," Deja said softly.

I walked into the bathroom and turned on the water to begin warming it. As I searched through Elizabeth's drawers for her usual bath soap and some washcloths, I came across her makeup bag. Until today, I had never seen Elizabeth without makeup, so I grabbed it.

While I cleaned her body and changed her clothes, Deja did her makeup with the skill of a professional. By the time we were done, Elizabeth looked beautiful.

"You know, she told me that she regretted spending so much of her life worrying about what others thought of her," I told Deja. "It was eye-opening for me."

"She told me that I was beautiful. She really meant it, too—I could tell. I don't know if I believe that about myself, but she meant it," Deja mused.

I smiled. "I think she would want you to believe it, it's true."

As Deja packed up and said her goodbyes, I noticed that her eyes were wet. "She's special," Deja said.

"She's my role model. We can all learn a lot from Elizabeth."

I WALKED BACK INTO Elizabeth's room, expecting the calm feeling to hit me again. Something was off, though. The lemon scent was still in the air and the music was still playing, but a certain energy was gone. I knew without knowing that Elizabeth was gone. Although it's hard to explain, this shift is one that every hospice nurse and person who has witnessed a death has experienced—the tangible shift in the air in that moment when a person leaves their body. It's not unlike when you walk into a room expecting someone to be there, only to discover you're alone. Sometimes that shift is more pronounced than others, and sometimes this moment occurs before their physical death, while other times it's after. In Elizabeth's case, her absence was very pronounced.

I pulled out my stethoscope and held it to Elizabeth's still chest, listening for a heartbeat that I knew wasn't there. After two minutes, I quietly spoke her time of death to the empty room. Elizabeth had left this world exactly as she had lived in it—alone.

YEARS LATER, I STILL think about Elizabeth. I remember how I never once saw her sad or angry, despite the fact that she died so young and so alone. She never asked, *Why me?* She was the very essence of making the most of what we're given.

Unbeknownst to her, Elizabeth also opened up an important conversation between Chris and me. Chris had no idea that I thought he wouldn't love me anymore if I didn't stay as skinny as I was when we met. In retrospect, *of course* he didn't think that, but the correlation of love and weight had been modeled to me from such a young age that I hadn't been able to untangle them . . . until I met Elizabeth.

Her words changed me: *Eat the cake.* Since then, every time I am on the brink of bingeing or purging, I hear those words. And, every time, they stop me and remind me of what really matters most.

Edith

"HEY, DO YOU HAVE TIME TO EVALUATE SOMEONE'S eligibility today?" Travis asked me.

"Yes, sure," I told him. These admission evaluations were a normal part of my routine. While it's a patient's physician who refers them to hospice, the patient also has to meet the eligibility requirements dictated by Medicare—the specifics of which doctors who don't specialize in hospice aren't always aware of. Hospice nurses are responsible for determining whether or not a patient is admissible according to Medicare's guidelines (which are based on very specific markers), and then running their determination by a certified physician for official approval—in our case, these approvals came from Dr. Kumar.

"Great," Travis continued. "Her name is Edith and she has Alzheimer's. She lives with her husband, John, and it seems like she's right on the line of being eligible for hospice."

"Got it," I said, already typing the address into my GPS.

EDITH AND JOHN'S HOUSE looked like it was out of a story-book. A pathway lined with bright pink flowers led up to a terra-cotta cottage covered in vines. As I pressed the doorbell, I heard commotion behind the door.

"*Please* just stay there for a moment, Edith," I heard a pleading voice say. A few seconds later, a short, white-haired man in his eighties answered the door, his back hunched over. "Come on, I can't leave her for long," he said by way of greeting.

As I walked in the house, I admired the beautiful antiques and weathered hardwood floors. The hallway was lined with family photos from a happier time. Clearly, this family had been adventurous—there were pictures of John and Edith and their kids in front of the Eiffel Tower, the Great Wall of China, and the Statue of Liberty. Beyond the hallway a tall woman with white hair, who also appeared to be in her eighties, was standing next to the couch in the living room. It was clear that she was the same woman as the one in those photos, just an older version, her once long, sandy brown hair now cut into a white-tinted bob. John and Edith's running shoes had been replaced with house slippers, but I could see from the photos that the wrinkles around their eyes and mouths came from many years of smiling.

"I told you not to get up. Please sit down!" John said to Edith, who towered at least a foot over him. He grabbed her hand and guided her down to the couch, clearly exasperated.

"Hi, my name is Hadley. I'm assuming you're Ms. Edith and Mr. John?" I asked.

"Yes, we are," John replied. Edith hummed incomprehensibly and looked out the window.

"I was told to evaluate Edith to see if she's eligible for hospice. Is that correct?"

"It is. I need some help. This has been going on for years," John replied. It was abundantly clear that he was exhausted and frustrated, which made perfect sense. I knew from our notes that John had been in this position for years. It's relentlessly taxing and tiring to be a caregiver—especially when Alzheimer's is involved. A patient's descent into dementia generally lasts for an extended period of time, until the caregiver ultimately finds themself in charge of an adult who relies on them for every single task.

I nodded while pulling out my stethoscope to get Edith's vital signs. There are different hospice eligibility scales for different diseases, and dementia patients are measured against the Functional Assessment Staging Tool, better known as the FAST Scale. Since Alzheimer's is progressive, the stages that the FAST Scale measures usually happen in sequence as a patient gradually declines. For admission into hospice, Alzheimer's patients need to score at least a 6E (moderately severe dementia) or 7A (severe dementia). Practically, this means that the patient can no longer go to the bathroom by themselves or speak more than five to six words in a given day. Sometimes, other elements of the patient's condition can be taken into consideration as well, such as falling, weight loss, and frequent or significant visits to the hospital.

I started evaluating Edith at number 4, mild dementia, which is usually when loved ones start to notice that something is going on and begin to intervene. "Is she having trouble doing things independently, such as paying bills or cooking meals?" I asked John. I could predict the answer, but had to ask anyway.

John looked at me like I was stupid. "Honey, she lost those abilities years ago."

I marked the categories 1 through 4, then moved down to 5, moderate dementia. "Do you have to help her choose her clothes? For example, would she know to put on shorts today since it's warm outside?"

"I definitely need to help her," John replied. I moved down to 6A through 6C, moderately severe dementia.

"Do you also need to help her get dressed?"

"Yes."

"What about bathing and going to the toilet?" I asked.

"Yes to bathing, and she wears Depends."

I checked yes to 6A through 6C, then moved down to 6D and 6E. "Does she need Depends all the time, or can she sometimes tell you when she needs to go to the bathroom?"

"She hasn't been to the bathroom in ages and she never asks to go. I just change her Depends when I smell them. Like a baby," he said bluntly.

I checked 6D and 6E, then moved down to 7A, severe dementia. If she had 7A then Dr. Kumar almost always said that I could admit the patient. "About how many comprehensible words does she speak in a day?" I asked.

"Maybe ten to twenty."

I nodded, unable to check that box.

As I scrolled down my list, Edith spoke for the first time. "The laundry," she said before swiftly—but unsteadily—getting up and walking toward the hallway. John got up quickly to stop her.

"God damn it, Edith. Sit down," he said. She looked at him, wide-eyed.

"I can do your laundry, Ms. Edith," I tried.

Edith looked at me, and then began aggressively shaking her head from side to side, trying to break free from John's grasp. He groaned in frustration. "Every second of every day," he said.

I looked around the room and spotted the basket of laundry on the dining room table, just off the hallway. As John held her steady, I went over and grabbed it, placing it on the floor next to the couch. Edith sat back on the couch and began picking up the laundry and folding it, examining each piece of clothing as she went. John sat down next to her, clearly exhausted from caregiving.

I continued down my admission checklist. "How is her eating?" I asked.

"Bad. She eats like a little bird, pecking at food. She has lost eleven pounds in the last two months," he replied, sounding defeated.

"I noticed that she's unsteady on her feet. Has she fallen at all?"

"I've lost track of how many times she's fallen. I can't even go to the bathroom anymore."

"Would you say more than ten times in the past month?"

"More like in the past week."

"Okay," I said. "I think I can go ahead and call our doctor now. Can I step outside for a moment?" John made a sweeping motion toward the front door with his arm as if to say, "Be my guest." I stepped out, tablet still in hand, and dialed Dr. Kumar's phone number.

"Hi, Hadley," he greeted me, sounding chipper as always.

"Okay," I started, "so I have an Alzheimer's patient for potential admit, but they are 6E. I think you might still be okay with admitting her, though."

"Hit me," he said.

"Her husband said she speaks between ten and twenty comprehensible words per day, and I did hear her say 'the laundry' in the correct context while I've been here, but she's lost eleven pounds in the last two months and is falling all the time, like more than ten times per week."

Dr. Kumar was quiet, and I knew he was considering the situation.

"Her husband really needs help. Please," I tried.

"You know it has to be objective, Hadley."

I stopped talking, nervous that he was going to tell me no.

"Go ahead and admit her," Dr. Kumar continued, "but we need to show decline in the first ninety days. I need strong charting, okay?"

"Yes, got it! Thank you," I told Dr. Kumar before hanging up and stepping back inside the home.

"Good news," I called out to John as I shut the door behind me. "We're good to admit."

"Great! I have some errands to run. I'll be back in a few hours," John said.

I paused, making sure to choose my words carefully. "I'm not sure if you were given inaccurate information, but we don't stay around the clock," I said gently. "I would encourage you to get more help, though. Our social worker can assist with paid caregivers or help place Ms. Edith in a nursing home–like setting."

John sighed, exasperated. "I promised her I wouldn't leave her, and I surely don't want her to go into a nursing home. How much are caregivers?"

"From what I've heard, about thirty dollars an hour, and they require a minimum number of hours each visit. Usually six hours or more."

"Thirty dollars an hour!" he exclaimed.

I nodded slowly. I understood how difficult it was to afford necessary care on a fixed income, but there weren't many other options. "What we do in hospice is come and help you care for Edith. For example, I'll start by coming once or twice per week, a nurse's aide will come two or three times a week to help her shower or bathe, our social worker comes about once a month, as well as our chaplain, and then there is always a nurse on call for any emergencies," I explained. "And if you *do* want to look into nursing home options, I wouldn't blame you."

John cut me off sharply, shaking his head from side to side. "Absolutely not. I'll make do."

Many people don't think about the fact that hospice and nursing home care are a business (I don't like thinking about it myself, honestly)—but they are. And if the costs aren't covered, they can be exorbitant and leave both the patient and their caregiver without any good options. Caregiving is hard, emotional, exhausting work that can go on for an extended period of time, much like it had been for John. Even with Medicare covering the cost of a hospice nurse like me, the caregiver is still in charge of the day-to-day care of the patient—which can be a lot. So, while I wanted to give John good news, the truth is that there really *aren't* a lot of options for people like him and Edith. Even if he had been open to the idea, you basically have to be really rich or really poor to afford a nursing home (because, in the latter case, the government steps in). There aren't many options in between—with the exception of hiring a caregiver, which is also expensive— and most people are in between.

I thought about all of this, but what I said was simply, "No problem." After completing the rest of the admission process and giving John the on-call nurse's number, I said goodbye to Edith, who was folding a washcloth for the third time.

She replied incomprehensibly and smiled as I touched her shoulder.

THE NEXT MORNING, I hurriedly applied my makeup as I listened to the on-hold music playing through the speaker on my phone, waiting for the daily meeting to start. We held this meeting every Monday through Friday so that the night and on-call nurses could update us about what had happened the night before.

"Good morning, everyone!" Travis greeted us. "Amanda, I'll let you take over. It sounds like your on-call night was eventful."

"Yes, um, I spent a lot of time at our new patient's home."

Uh-oh, I thought, *here we go.* "Ms. Edith fell twice so I went out to assess her and make sure she was okay. Her vital signs were good and her mental status seemed to be at her baseline."

I let out a breath. Okay, this wasn't an unusual on-call night. Things like this happened all the time.

"So, I got her calm and back in bed and went home," Amanda continued. "And then, about an hour later, I got another call from her husband. Ms. Edith had gotten out of the house and he couldn't find her."

I placed my blush down and sat on the toilet.

"I drove around helping John look for her for a few minutes, and then we ended up calling the police to help. They eventually found Ms. Edith in a ditch about a quarter mile away from her home, picking at the grass. She was unharmed."

"Hadley, you need to get with Mindy this morning and plan to go to their home today. This is unsafe. She needs to go into a nursing home," Travis said. Mindy was the social worker for whenever our patients needed additional assistance, including things like helping them with insurance and accessing additional programs outside of regular hospice services.

"John was adamant that he wouldn't put her there, but I understand," I said. I muted the phone and let out a deep sigh. I hated being in situations like this.

LATER THAT MORNING, I was back at the cottage, this time with Mindy by my side, psyching myself up for what I knew was going to be a tough conversation. But when the front door swung open, we were greeted by a man who looked like he was ready to wave a white flag.

"Hey, John, this is Mindy, our social worker," I said in greeting. I was dismayed to see that John looked even more hunched over than he had yesterday. Edith was sitting on the couch, still in her pajamas. She had a TV tray in front of her with a plate full of waffles that she was picking up and placing down again, but not eating. Children's cartoons played on the TV across the room from her, keeping her entertained for the time being.

"We heard about last night," Mindy began gently. "I wanted to tell you about some of the benefits of full-time assistance."

"Just put us somewhere and forget about us," John said, sounding defeated. "I died long ago when she lost all memories of us."

I felt as if a dagger was stabbing me in the heart. I couldn't imagine the pain of caring for someone you loved who didn't recognize you on most days. I had no idea how to respond.

"Well, here's some options," Mindy continued, placing a piece of paper on the coffee table in front of us. "They really are lovely facilities. State-of-the-art." I attempted to read upside-down the typed-up list of all of the nursing homes and assisted-living facilities nearby that had locked units. Below each facility name, Mindy had included the estimated monthly cost. The prices ranged from $8,750 to $11,000 per month.

"We'll run out of money in a few years, but we could do ten thousand per month for both of us," he said.

"That price is actually just for one of you," Mindy replied.

A stream of curse words flew from John's mouth. "We can only afford one of us, so what are our other options?" he asked.

Mindy and I traded looks, knowing there really *were* no other options.

John must have picked up on what we were thinking. "Okay, I understand. I'll think about it. *If* I choose this, which is the best one?" he asked us.

"We aren't technically allowed to share our opinions. I'm sorry," Mindy replied.

I bit my lip to keep from speaking; I wanted to share my opinion so badly. I had strong feelings about how each of these facilities treated their patients.

John sighed and put his head in his hands. "I'm on my own like usual, then. Got it."

Mindy gave me a look as she began packing up her bag. She knew I was going to share my opinions as soon as she walked out the door, and I knew she didn't really care.

As soon as I heard the door shut, I turned back toward John. He was sitting on the couch with the list of nursing homes in his hands. He spoke before I could. "I've heard great things about Sutton Heights," he said.

I let out an audible sigh of relief that I wasn't going to have to put myself in a situation where I could get into trouble. Sutton Heights was my absolute favorite. The nurses had worked there forever, they were great about communicating with me, and I never had concerns about how they treated their patients. I started nodding my head up and down aggressively, figuring that was okay. John looked up at me quizzically and then he smiled, like this was a game.

"What about Beach View?" he said. I stopped nodding, widened my eyes, and sucked my lips in, not saying anything yet saying everything.

John laughed. "Sutton Heights, got it," he said with a genuine smile.

I smiled back at him, and finally exhaled. "So, should we go ahead and get the paperwork for Sutton Heights going?"

"No, I'm not ready yet," John said, suddenly stern again.

I bit my lip, knowing Travis would be upset, but unsure what else to do. John had a right to keep his wife at home, even if we didn't necessarily agree with the decision.

"Okay," I said, shrugging. "Let's do our absolute best here, then."

"That easy, huh?" John asked.

"I'm here to help you and Edith. Y'all are in the driver's seat. I'm in the backseat; you can either ask me for directions or tell me to keep quiet," I said with a smile.

"Okay, I've got this," he said confidently.

I wish I could say this is when things got easier for him.

A FEW WEEKS LATER, I got a frantic phone call in the middle of the night. "Hi, this is Edith's husband, John. Um, I don't know how to describe what's going on," he said as soon as I picked up the phone. "I think you need to come over here."

I could hear commotion in the background. It sounded like Edith was . . . yelling? "Is she in pain?" I asked.

"She thinks the bedroom's on fire," John told me, sounding exhausted.

When I arrived, John and Edith were in their bedroom. John was sitting on the bed trying to orient Edith, but she was not having it. She paced back and forth and back and forth, mumbling to herself and randomly shouting "Fire!" over and over again. I had already called Dr. Kumar on the way over and he instructed me to give Edith the emergency anti-anxiety medications that we had ordered when she was first admitted.

For the next ten minutes I tried to calm Edith down, to no

avail. She continued to pace, pull at her hair, and say that the room was on fire. I called Dr. Kumar again, and this time he instructed me to give her another dose of the anti-anxiety meds and try to distract her. I did as he told me and offered to get Edith some food, but she shook her head no. John tried to give her some food, but she pushed it away. I went into the living room and turned on the TV. Popping my head back into the bedroom, I asked her to come watch with me. She sat down on the bed, continuing to tell me that it was on fire, tears now running down her face.

Thirty minutes in, I was starting to panic, and all three of us were distressed. I finally pulled out my phone and dialed the number of a veteran nurse who'd been doing this job for more than fifteen years.

"Hello?" Linda answered groggily in her British accent.

"It's Hadley," I said, cringing. "I'm so sorry to call out of the blue and in the middle of the night, please don't be mad. I have a patient with Alzheimer's who thinks her bed is on fire. She's just pacing and crying. I've given her two doses of anti-anxiety medication, but it's not working *at all*," I hurriedly explained.

"Love, why don't you move her bedroom elsewhere?" Linda asked.

"Uh, I'm sorry—what does that even mean?" I replied, confused.

"Where is the fire?"

"Well, there's no real fire."

"Now, now dear, to her there *is* a fire. It's on her bed, right? That's distressing. Why don't you move her bed away from the fire so she can go to sleep?" Linda coached.

"Linda, I don't think that's going to work."

"Try it first, and call me back if it doesn't work. But I bet you that it does. Nighty night," she said, hanging up the phone.

I stared at Edith and John's full-size bed. How would I move it and where would I even put it? I beckoned John over. "I called a nurse who has a ton of experience. She thinks I should move y'all's bed away from the 'fire.' I know it seems crazy, but is there a different bedroom I could move it to, by chance?"

John, clearly exhausted, got up and opened the door to a bedroom just down the hall that was completely empty.

"Okay, that definitely works. Um, is it okay if I move your bed?" I asked.

"You are about the strangest backseat driver I've ever had, but I trust you for some reason. Go ahead." I went back into the bedroom and assessed the bed, trying to figure out the best way to move it. It looked like it would fit out the wide double-door without having to be disassembled. Edith stood by my side as I looked at the bed, as if she was assessing it too. A few moments later, she let out a weak whimper as she said, yet again, "Fire." This was too much. It broke my heart to see her in so much distress. I was just going to have to go for it.

Walking up to the heavy-looking wooden bed, I attempted to pull it out from the wall. Surprisingly, the wood must have been fake; the bed easily slid over the carpet and toward me. I now had enough room to shimmy between the back of the headboard and the wall. I started pushing the bed across the carpet, peering out every few seconds to make sure I was still heading in the right direction. Once I was about halfway out of their bedroom, Edith came up next to me and started pushing too. I'm not sure if she knew what we were doing, and she surely didn't contribute much to the bed actually moving, but I smiled at her as we pushed it toward the hallway side by side. Once we got it into the other bedroom, I stopped and looked around, trying to decide where to put the bed. Edith pointed to the back left corner of the room.

"There?" I asked her.

She nodded adamantly in response.

I obliged, pushing the bed until it was in that corner of the room. To my complete surprise, as soon as I pushed the bed into place and stood back, Edith crawled into it and seemed to go to sleep. It had actually worked! I was shocked.

"Good job," John whispered, once the two of us were confident that Edith was sleeping soundly. I placed my hand on his shoulder and smiled at him.

"You've got this. You're doing a good job," I assured him.

"It's time," he said. "Let Sutton Heights know she's coming."

I nodded. Tonight had been difficult. I knew John was making the right intellectual decision, but I worried about his heart.

LESS THAN A WEEK later, I was walking through the glass doors at Sutton Heights.

"Ms. Edith?" the young receptionist asked me.

"Yes. Have you met her yet?"

"Her husband practically lives here. I've let him in the locked unit quite a few times already," she said.

"I am not surprised one bit. Do you mind making that trip once more?"

The receptionist stepped out from behind the desk and led me back to the locked unit, entering the code that opened the heavy doors.

"I call it Hotel California," she said, waiting for the doors to click open.

"Huh?" I asked, confused.

"You can check in any time you want, but you can never leave."

The receptionist's words unsettled me. A loud buzzing interrupted my thoughts and I quickly stepped inside the unit. As I approached the nurses' station, I spotted the unit manager, one of my favorite nurses there.

"Hey!" I greeted her.

"Who ya got today?" she asked, knowing I had quite a few patients on the unit.

Before I could respond, I felt a hand on my back. I turned to see another one of my patients. She started petting my hair as I smiled at her. "Your new one. I had her at home," I told the nurse while feeling my hair being lifted away from my face then falling back down. It would be odd in any other context, but it was by no means out of the ordinary for us.

"Ah, yes, Edith. She's doing great! She participated in dance class earlier. She's in room six."

"Oh my gosh, I wish I could have seen it!" I smiled. With that, I told the patient petting my hair that I had to go, but I would see her tomorrow. She mumbled back to me incomprehensibly, but smiled, so I took that as an "okay." I walked down the brightly lit hallway to room six. John opened the door, and for the first time since I'd met him he looked well rested. In the room, Edith rocked in a chair near a window that overlooked the garden. She smiled at me as I walked in.

"How's it going?" I asked, almost scared to hear John's answer.

"Actually, really well," he said, smiling at Edith. Edith smiled back at him. Relieved, I pulled out my blood pressure cuff to start my assessment. "I have to run an errand. Is that okay with you?"

"Absolutely! Don't stress if you're not always here. I can always get a report from the nurses and call to update you."

"Well, I don't know if I'll loosen the reins that easily, but thank you for the offer," John said before kissing Edith on the forehead and leaving the room.

I continued through my questions while Edith stared out at the garden, watching the birds and butterflies fly by her window. When I reached the question asking for her weight, I told Edith I'd be right back, since I needed to ask the nurse for the answer.

Out in the hallway, I could hear what sounded like arguing. "If you don't let me out of here right this second, you'll be hearing from my lawyers!" a man was yelling.

"Sir, maybe we could just play some cards?" a scrub-clad employee pleaded with the man, who I could now see was John.

"I'm not confused, you crazy lady! I'm just going home!" John yelled back at her.

"This is your home. You're safe here," the sweet employee tried.

My walk turned into a jog as I realized that she thought John was a confused patient trying to escape.

"Hey, I know him. He's one of my patients' husband. He's not a patient here," I told her.

"Oh! Oh, my gosh. I'm so sorry, sir. I'm new," she said to John as she entered the code to unlock the door. As soon as he exited and the heavy door clanged behind him, I couldn't help but giggle. The employee looked scared.

"You did nothing wrong, it's your job. You're doing a good job. He'll get over it, I promise you," I reassured her, trying to suppress my giggles. I went back into Edith's room and completed my assessment while telling her the story. Edith laughed with me, as if she understood.

AS THE MONTHS WENT on, Ms. Edith gradually declined, but she never had any pain or any other episodes of anxiety. Over time, she went from being able to speak twenty words to under ten, to fewer than five, to just one word: "John."

Then she lost her ability to walk. That day was hard for everyone, including the nursing home staff, who had come to love Edith—but especially for John. He continued to come to the nursing home every single day, learning to transfer his wife to a wheelchair. He wheeled her out for meals so they could eat together in the dining room and she could get a change of scenery. And then, gradually, Edith lost the ability to sit up straight in her wheelchair, so John placed a pillow between her arm and the hard metal of the wheelchair to help hold her upright. She always looked up at him and smiled, even though she could no longer communicate with him.

There wasn't a specific day when Edith stopped smiling; it was more of a gradual thing. John pointed it out to me.

"I noticed that," I told him. "Unfortunately, it's part of the expected stages."

"Not being able to smile anymore is a stage of Alzheimer's?" John asked, looking shocked.

"Do you want me to be up-front with you?" I asked him.

"Yes, I don't want surprises."

I pulled out my tablet to show John the table that I had memorized by this point.

"We started here," I showed him, "and now we're here." I slid my finger down the chart from 6E to 7E.

"So, the last stage is being unable to hold up her own head?"

I nodded, grimacing.

"This is such a cruel disease," John sighed, shaking his head in disbelief.

"It is. It really is," I agreed.

AS THE MONTHS PASSED, I expected John's visits to slow, but he never missed a day. In Edith's last month of life, she was unable to get out of bed. I started coming more often, always checking on her when I had other patients at Sutton Heights, even if I wasn't scheduled to see her that day.

One day I walked in and noticed Edith's body was in an unnatural position. I walked farther into the room and saw tears rolling down her face. As I tried to talk to her and rub her back, I realized she was in extreme pain. I quickly ran out to get the nurse.

"Do you have those emergency medications on hand?" I asked urgently.

"I have to put a pain number in the computer to give the medicine. What should I put?" the nurse asked me.

"It's a ten. Labored breathing, crying, facial grimacing, fists clenched, tense, and unable to console." The nurse plugged the number in and handed me the medication.

"Nothing's been wrong with her?" I asked.

"No, nothing," she confirmed.

After giving the medication a few minutes to work and seeing Edith's body relax, I started assessing her, beginning at her head, as always. Her pupils were equal in size. I noticed no cuts or scrapes around her face or scalp. Her hair was nicely braided and looked freshly washed.

"Can you tell me your name?" I asked, knowing she wouldn't answer and checking the box that she wasn't oriented-to-self before moving down the list.

"Can you tell me where you are right now?" I asked. No response.

"Do you know what month it is?" I asked, while simultaneously checking the box indicating that she wasn't oriented to time.

"Hadley," I heard, loud and clear. I looked up from my tablet, expecting to see the Sutton Heights nurse. No one was there. I looked around, confused before looking down at Edith, who was looking directly at me. There was no way she just said my name. Her disease wouldn't allow her to remember me, much less be able to say my name.

"Hadley," she said once more, still looking up at me.

"Yes, that's me," I told her, reaching out to hold her hand. "I'm your nurse. I've been your nurse for quite some time now. I'm taking care of you. You're going to be okay. I promise."

Maybe it was a muscle spasm or maybe it was Edith's way of communicating with me (although she shouldn't have been able to), but her hand squeezed mine for just a moment. As I held my tablet in one hand and Edith's hand in the other, she slowly drifted off to sleep.

Glad that she was pain-free, I moved on to assessing her skin. I looked at her arms and legs. They were slightly bruised, as most elderly people's arms and legs are, but otherwise perfectly fine. While moving Edith onto her left side, I assessed her back. I audibly gasped as I pulled down her shorts. The largest and deepest pressure ulcer that I had ever seen had formed just above her bottom. It was larger than my fist, pear-shaped, and purple, black, and red all at the same time.

I felt my face heat up with rage. In school, I learned that pressure ulcers usually form as a result of not turning a patient as often as they needed to be turned. Letting them sit in one position for too long creates pressure on the area and causes the skin to break down. I felt angry and embarrassed that I had recommended this facility and they had let my patient down. I dreaded having to tell John.

I called Travis because I was unsure how to handle informing the facility of their neglect. As soon as he answered, I told him about the gaping wound that the nursing home didn't seem to know anything about.

"Wait, I don't think this is what you think it is. Hold on," he said. Confused, I waited as I heard him typing.

"Deja was there last night and reported that Ms. Edith's skin only had minimal bruising on her legs and arms," he said. After a pause, Travis asked, "Have you ever heard of a Kennedy ulcer?"

"No," I responded, thinking back to my wound care class in nursing school.

"So, you know how the skin is an organ, correct?"

"Yes," I said, unsure where he was going with this.

"Well, just like our organs start to shut down at the end of life, our skin can too. Kennedy ulcers can appear quite literally out of nowhere and look absolutely horrible. No one did anything wrong. You just need to ensure she isn't in pain because of it."

I had never heard of a Kennedy ulcer, but I was glad Travis had told me before I embarrassed myself and wrongfully accused the nursing home staff of wrongdoing. The relief I felt quickly turned to dread when I realized that I had to call John and prepare him for what was going to come next. With slightly shaking hands, I clicked John's number on my phone. He answered cheerfully.

"Hey, have you been by Sutton Heights yet today?" I asked him hesitantly.

"Nope, I'm on my way, though!"

"Okay, I'll stay and we can talk then," I told him.

As I waited, I observed Edith and made sure she wasn't uncomfortable. I wished that she could tell me what she was seeing in her dreams.

A short while later, John walked in and immediately went to her side. "Something is different," he said, looking concerned. I was surprised but impressed that he noticed. He was so in tune with his wife. I placed my hand on his shoulder and began explaining to him what had happened since I had arrived. John cried silently as he listened.

"I feel so foolish saying this, but I'm not ready. You would think that, with everything we've been through, this wouldn't be shocking to me," he said, wiping his nose with a tissue.

"I think that's normal."

"So, what's next?"

"I'm going to spend some time educating the nursing home staff so they know when to give her medicine again and when to call us. Then, if I'm not needed in the middle of the night, I'll see y'all again tomorrow. Is that okay with you?"

"Yes. And thanks for everything, Hadley," he said.

THERE WERE NO PHONE calls about Edith that night—or any other night, for that matter. I visited Edith and John every day for the next five days until she passed. I wasn't there when it happened, but I was told that it was very peaceful.

Much to my surprise, John had already left by the time I arrived at the facility about twenty minutes after Edith died. The nurse let me know that he couldn't handle seeing her like that.

I cleaned Edith up, talking to her the whole time, and then opened up the window overlooking the garden. As I waited for the funeral home to arrive, I watched the butterflies and birds flit past just as Ms. Edith had done a few months prior. When the funeral home workers arrived, I told Edith good-bye one last time before they placed the sheet over her face. I always look away before they do that—it's my least favorite moment. I panic every time, thinking that they can't breathe, even though I know it's a nonsensical fear.

After I completed all of my documentation and made all

my phone calls, I said goodbye to the Sutton Heights staff before continuing on with my day.

I was in my office half-heartedly doing paperwork when our chaplain, Steve, came in and sat down next to me. "I talked to Chris today," he said. Steve often went into the nursing home where Chris worked to see hospice patients, and he and Chris had developed a close relationship over the years. In fact, they'd known each other longer than I'd known either of them.

"Oh, yeah?" I asked.

"Yeah. We talked about his mom. We prayed for her."

"Oh, that's so sweet of you. Thank you so much for that."

"She says she's going to beat cancer," Steve said, looking at me.

I pursed my lips, not saying anything and looking straight at my computer. I knew better. I took care of lots of patients with brain cancer.

"You don't think so, I'm guessing," he said.

I shook my head very slightly.

"I think you might be a bit biased," he said, challenging me in a way I had not been challenged before. Most people tiptoed very delicately around Babette's illness and impending death.

"I've never had a patient beat brain cancer," I told him flatly.

"You only take care of people in the last stages of life, Hadley. She isn't there yet. I don't think it would hurt to think positively," he offered nonjudgmentally.

All of my feelings bubbled up to the surface at once, feelings that, until this moment, I had kept well concealed. "I can't be positive about this. Death sucks and it's everywhere. I get close to my patients, and then they die. I get off work and we go see Babette and just looking at her is a constant reminder. We don't go on any long trips, just in case. We aren't moving forward with our lives and getting engaged because it just seems wrong right now. There's a heaviness in the air every holiday because everyone's thinking it's probably her last, but no one's saying it," I said, my heart racing. I don't think I had ever shared those feelings with anyone. I didn't feel worthy of these feelings. Every time I felt them, I was reminded of how much worse everyone else had it; at least I wasn't dying.

"You know it's okay to feel like that, right?" Steve asked gently. "It's completely normal."

"I took the same courses as you and I also learned to tell people that their feelings are normal. That doesn't work on me," I told him, before bursting into laughter, which quickly turned into tears. I wasn't expecting this release of emotion, but getting all of it off my chest made me feel so much better.

"I have friends who are therapists. I could give you their numbers, you know," he said to me with fatherly concern.

"I promise I'm more okay than I seem right now," I said, wiping away my tears and thanking him for taking the time to listen.

THE WINTER PASSED, AS did many more patients under my care. You know that first day when the weather is in the high sixties, the sun is shining, the birds are chirping, and you can just feel spring coming to lift off the heavy weight of winter? It was on one of those perfect days when I walked up to the locked doors at Sutton Heights, waiting to be let inside. As I waited, a brightly colored flyer affixed to the door caught my eye.

It read TRIBUTE TO EDITH. There was going to be a small ceremony in the facility's garden, during which a bench would be placed there in her memory. I quickly searched for the date and time so I could make sure to be there, only to realize that the ceremony was today—and, in fact, it was happening right that very moment. I walked toward the doors that led out to the garden, and quietly joined the group that was listening to John tell stories about Edith. He held an urn in his hand as he shared how he had spent the last few months traveling to their favorite destinations and spreading Edith's ashes. He looked happy, and I was happy for him. After he finished, John spread a few of her ashes by the bench.

Afterward, I waited while well-wishers walked up to John, hugging him and patting him on the back. When I saw him notice me, I waved.

"Hadley, I'm so glad you're here!" he exclaimed. "I wanted to call you, but I don't want you to think I'm some crazy old man."

"John, I would never think that about you," I assured him. "You are absolutely welcome to call me anytime. I should have told you that." I worried that I hadn't made myself open and available to a grieving family member.

"No, no. Not like that. I have a story to tell you! I don't think anyone else would understand it like you, but you might also think I'm crazy." John's eyes lit up as he spoke; I had never seen him like this before. He was even standing up straighter, a completely new man.

"I promise not to think you're crazy," I assured him. At this point, I didn't think anything could really surprise me.

"Do you remember when Edith thought the bedroom was on fire?" he asked.

"Of course. I'll never forget it," I told him sincerely.

"Well, they aren't really sure what happened, possibly an electrical fire, but that bedroom caught on fire one night a few months after Edith died," he said, excited.

I'm sure my face showed my shock. It took me a minute to slow my racing thoughts and respond. "Are you okay?" I asked, figuring that was the most appropriate question.

"Yes, but only because I never moved the bed back. I've been sleeping in that extra bedroom ever since you moved the bed." John paused for a moment before confidently saying, "Edith knew."

My brain reached for any other possible conclusion, but I couldn't find one. "I guess she did," I said slowly.

But . . . *how* could she have known?

ALTHOUGH I HAD SEEN many puzzling and surprising things by this point in my hospice career, this was the first incident that struck me as truly inexplicable. And yet, also, undismissable. I'm sure that someone might argue that this fire Edith had apparently foreseen was a coincidence—but that's an awfully big coincidence, and an unsatisfactory explanation from my point of view.

My experience with Edith made me think about Alzheimer's patients differently from that point on. It's easy to focus on the fact that, in so many ways, they don't seem to be here anymore. But what we don't think about as often is: *Where are they?* I often refer to my patients as having one foot on this side and one on the other. But I now suspect—although I obviously can't prove—that while they're still physically here, beyond a certain point Alzheimer's patients are more firmly planted in whatever place we go next, on the other side. It can be easy to look at them as if they're toddlers, almost like they don't know what's going on. And yet, I don't think that's the case at all. Edith—and many other dementia patients I've worked with over the years—have defied that assumption, doing things that, from a scientific or medical perspective, they shouldn't be able to do.

How did Edith know my name—let alone say it—when she was that deep in her diagnosis, long after she had lost the cognitive ability to form new memories? How did she know precisely where the fire was going to happen? I look at and treat my patients with my nursing brain, but my nursing brain can't explain these things. I believe in medicine and science, but my own experience tells me that, while they can explain a lot, they can't explain everything.

To this day, I can't explain why or how all of this happened. I just know that it did.

Shortly after John told me about the fire, I ran into Linda, the nurse who had advised me to move Edith's bed the night when I thought she was hallucinating. I told her what had happened, and she seemed unsurprised.

"That stuff happens," she said simply, shrugging her shoulders. "I'm glad you moved the bed."

Reggie

As I walked up to the restaurant, I saw my long-time friends already sitting at a bistro table outside, sipping wine. It was unusually warm for January, but I was still grateful to see that they had snagged a table by a heater.

"Hey guys!" I said as I plopped down in the empty chair across from Molly and next to Kelly.

"We were just talking about work," Molly said.

I nodded and smiled. Molly worked in retail sales. My other friend Kelly worked as a receptionist at a real estate office. As Kelly finished telling us a story about a client who was turned down for a mortgage and upset at her because of it, the waiter brought out my wine. "Cheers!" we chorused.

Picking up where we'd left off, Molly leaned in and said, "I totally get it. I had a customer the other day who got all worked up over a coupon not working. On top of that, I feel like every single person who came in made a complete mess of the clothing piles. I could barely get anything else done."

I nodded and munched on some cheese from the charcuterie board in the middle of the table.

"What about you, Hads? How's your job going?"

I tried to think of a way to respond. Somehow *I had a patient die this morning, and then listened to a soon-to-be widow cry over things out of her control this afternoon* didn't seem like the right topic for happy hour drinks with friends I wasn't able to see too often.

"Same old, same old," I said with a shrug, wishing that I could share the details of, and my feelings about, my job—but I knew it would bring down the mood. I shoved another piece of cheese in my mouth to indicate that I wasn't planning to elaborate.

This wasn't an uncommon situation, and it wasn't limited to my friends. In the past couple of years, I'd gotten into the habit of keeping work stories to myself. I loved my job, and the truth is that, despite the death I witnessed and the emotions that came with it, working in hospice made me feel more alive than I ever had before. It seemed clear to me that I had found my true calling in life. But, nonetheless, my line of work made other people uncomfortable.

I quickly grew accustomed to people changing the subject when I brought up the topic of my job in social situations, so I had gotten used to changing it myself. And, in the few times when I hadn't, I regretted that choice. When Chris and I had attended a charity event over the holidays, a doctor struck up a conversation that included asking both of us what we did for work. Chris shared that he was a physical therapist; when the doctor turned to me, I told him that I was a hospice nurse.

"Oh," he said, making a face as he swirled his drink in his hand. "That's depressing." And this was from a *doctor*.

"Not really," I replied, smiling. "I really enjoy it—"

"You *enjoy* death?" the doctor cut me off.

I felt my face heat up. "There's a lot more to it," I explained, feeling myself fumble over my words as I spoke. "It's not death all the time."

"Mmmm," he replied, clearly disengaged. "Well, it was lovely to meet you both." With that, he turned his back on us. I felt so embarrassed and wished I would have just said I was a nurse and left it at that.

Strangers weren't the only people who were confused by my job. Some of my friends and family were too, even when I explained how much the work meant to me. In one particularly painful conversation, my dad asked when I planned on going back to being a "real nurse." When I protested that I *was* a real nurse, he replied, "Well, a nurse that actually does stuff to save lives instead of just letting patients die."

Much as I tried to shove it down, that conversation kept replaying in my head. A few nights later, Chris's parents asked how my job was going over dinner. Feeling defeated, I responded differently than I usually did.

"It's okay," I said with a half smile.

Chris looked surprised. "You love your job!" he protested.

"I know," I said, looking down at my dinner plate. "But sometimes I second-guess it. Maybe it would be better if I went back to the hospital."

"Someone told Hadley that she wasn't a real nurse," Chris bluntly told his parents. He continued talking, but Babette interrupted.

"Hadley," she said, looking me directly in the eye, "does your job make you happy?"

"It does." I shrugged.

"Then that's all that matters," Babette said firmly, as if the matter was settled. "Life is short—don't I know it! And if your happiness doesn't affect anyone else, well, then screw 'em! They don't get a say in the matter."

To this day, I hold that moment close to my heart.

Molly and Kelly didn't seem to notice that I was being evasive, though, and the conversation quickly turned to relationships.

"Well, Brooks and I finally picked out a venue!" Molly said.

I smiled and exhaled, relieved about the change of subject. I listened happily as she filled us in on all the details about their wedding venue.

"What about you two? Any wedding bells soon?" Molly asked, turning to me.

Chris and I had looked at rings a few months ago, but he hadn't mentioned it since. I would be lying if I said I wasn't a little disappointed, but Babette was so sick and I knew she needed to be the focus right now.

"I'm ready and waiting!" Kelly joked.

"Me too!" I agreed in earnest.

We finished up and paid our bill, promising to see each other very soon. From there, I headed over to the beach, where I knew Chris had taken Brody after picking him up from daycare so that I could spend a little bit of time with my friends. There I spotted the two of them building a sandcastle off in the distance. With the wind whipping my hair around my face, I stopped for a moment and stared at the ocean as the waves rolled in. I knew that my patient who passed today would soon be replaced by a new patient. A never-ending cycle, as predictable as the ocean's tides. I wondered who I would be caring for next.

IT DIDN'T TAKE LONG to answer that question. A new admission was placed on my schedule two days later. I read the notes: *Reggie is a fifty-eight-year-old male with end-stage liver disease. Not a candidate for transplant due to alcohol consumption within the last six months. Wife's name is Lisa and she is his caregiver. They have no children or other support.* There was a handwritten note circled in red at the top of the page: *High deductible, charity?* And beneath that was scrawled the word *approved.*

I sighed in relief. Hospice is covered by Medicare, but it's more complicated for patients like Reggie who are not yet sixty-five years old. Sometimes private insurance will cover 100 percent of the hospice fees, but other times the patient needs to meet their deductible, which can be thousands of dollars. This charity approval—which was rare, accounting for only about 1 percent of our patients—meant that my company would cover all the costs that insurance wouldn't.

AS I SAT AT my desk reviewing the rest of Reggie's paperwork, I heard Steve's distinct voice. "Hey, hey, hey," he called out as he rounded the corner into the nurses' office. I swiveled in my chair to face him and smiled. He was dressed in a white button-down shirt and black slacks, both perfectly pressed. He swung a chair up next to me, the plastic wheels clamoring against the tile. "How's Babette?" he asked. "She's been in my prayers."

"Still losing weight. She has an oncologist here in town and she goes to MD Anderson every few months. Sometimes I feel like they push her off onto each other and no one is truly in charge, but, you know, she's a nurse and says she has it handled, so I don't want to overstep," I replied.

"*Does* she have it handled?" Steve asked.

I paused. Something about Steve allowed me to be honest.

I sighed heavily. "I don't know. She seems okay, but I've noticed she's doing little things, like forgetting the code to the storage unit. But we don't know if that's the cancer or something that could happen to anyone. I want the best for her, but I don't want to take away anything else from her."

Steve scooted his chair a little closer and leaned in before speaking. "Let me ask you this: If you don't intervene, what's the worst thing that could happen?"

"She wouldn't get the best treatment possible," I answered, feeling a little confused about his line of questioning.

"And what's the worst thing that would happen if you did intervene?"

"She might get better treatment, but she might not. Also, she would probably be hurt that I didn't let her handle it."

"I think you know what to do," he said with a reassuring pat on my arm, before walking toward the nearby kitchen.

I sighed and nodded, swiveling my chair back toward the mountain of admission paperwork.

"Who's that?" Steve asked, gesturing to my paperwork while pouring himself a cup of coffee.

"Reggie," I replied. "A possible new patient I'll be seeing very soon. I just read that he's an atheist, so I don't think they'll want a chaplain. But I'll offer your services just in case."

"I can offer any level of support they need. I won't talk about anything they don't want me to, okay?"

I smiled and shook my head. "I know, but most people don't believe me when I tell them that. They think you're going to show up with holy water and start throwing it on them."

"I won't even bring in my bottled drinking water. Cross my heart. Wait, no—no crosses. Pinky promise," Steve chuckled, offering his pinky to me.

I laughed and intertwined my pinky with his.

THAT AFTERNOON, I ARRIVED at Reggie's house—a trailer home in need of repairs. I noticed a man next door looking at me, holding a cigarette between his lips. I waved at him while walking through the dense grass up to Reggie's home, then yelped as my right foot stepped in a hole that wasn't visible. The neighbor laughed at my expense. I stepped out of the hole and finished my trek to the front door, where I rang the door-bell.

"Doesn't work, sweetheart," the neighbor yelled to me.

I knocked instead and was greeted by a loud bark.

"Oh, be quiet, Max," I heard someone say from behind the closed door. A moment later a woman wearing a plain black dress and who looked to be in her early fifties opened the door. Her black hair was tucked neatly behind her ears, but fell in front of her face as she leaned down to grab Max's collar.

"I am so sorry," she said as Max started to calm down. His fluffy tail wagged in true golden retriever fashion.

"I'm totally used to it," I said. "I'm Hadley. Nice to meet you."

"Lisa. Nice to meet you too. Reggie is right in here."

She led me into the living room, which was decorated with a faux leather sofa and a coffee table littered with magazines, cigarettes, and various takeout cups. The box TV that sat in an old wooden hutch was muted, but a daytime game show played on the screen. Directly across from the TV, Reggie sat in a recliner. He was wearing a plain white T-shirt and pajama pants that were stretched tight against his bloated stomach. This type of bloat is known as "ascites," and it's a hallmark symptom of liver cancer.

Lisa walked over and lightly shook Reggie to wake him up. He looked confused until his eyes landed on me. "You're finally fulfilling my dying wish, huh?" he asked his wife.

I was touched that he was so grateful for hospice, but his wife knew him better. "Don't even say it. I'm serious, Reggie," she said in a scolding tone.

"You got me my own personal stripper?" he said anyway, then laughed. My eyes widened. I had no idea how to respond. I glanced down at my outfit, and the same baggy blue scrubs and tennis shoes that I always wore stared back at me.

"He's confused," Lisa quickly said, trying to explain his words away. "It's part of the disease."

I nodded at her and ignored Reggie. A year ago, I would have excused such behavior, but I knew better now.

"I need to assess you to see if you're eligible for hospice. Is that okay?" I asked.

"Of course, we need help. We really appreciate you," Lisa answered before Reggie could speak again. I placed my nursing bag down and pulled out my tablet.

"Okay, first question. Can you tell me your name?"

"Reggie Bush. Can't you tell? I look just like him," Reggie replied with a grimace.

"I'm seeing a different last name," I said.

"Oh, you're no fun!" he sighed. "I'm used to these questions, I just got out of the hospital. My name is Reggie. It's January right now. What else do you need to know?"

I checked two of the three boxes indicating that he knew "person" and "time," but I needed to know if he knew "place."

"Do you know where you are right now?"

"Yeah: Hell," he replied flatly, then reached out to the table next to him to grab the sweating can of Bud Light. "I'm at my house," he sighed. "This is my wife, Lisa. This is my dog, Max. This is what got me here," he said, holding up the beer in a "cheers" motion before throwing his head back and finishing it off.

I checked the "place" box, indicating that he wasn't confused about where he was. I pulled out my penlight to start my physical assessment. I always started my examination at the top of the body, the head, and moved to the bottom, the toes, so I wouldn't miss a step. I walked closer to Reggie and noticed that the whites of his eyes were yellow—a sign of advanced liver disease. As I moved down Reggie's body, I saw that his arms were thin. The skin around them was loose, a grim reminder that he used to be muscular.

"What did you do for work?" I asked to fill the silence.

"Construction."

"I'm sure you stayed busy around here. I swear there's a new building going up every time I turn around."

"Everyone wants a piece of the beach," he said. "Lisa and I moved down here when it was still a small fishermen's village. There was nothing out here then. That's how we have this property. Every developer in town has tried to buy it from me, but I just tell them no, because even if I sell it for the hundreds of thousands they want to give me, where am I supposed to go? Everything else costs even more."

"They want us out of town, Reggie. That's the whole point," Lisa called out from the nearby kitchen. "They don't like trash like us."

"Well, don't you let them take it, Lisa. You hear me?"

"Who am I supposed to give it to, huh? We ain't got no kids and no family."

"Give it to her," he said, pointing to me with his beer as I pulled my measuring tape out of my nursing bag. Lisa rolled her eyes. It was clear to me that this was a regular disagreement between them that didn't seem to have a reasonable solution.

"I don't think your neighbor would like that," I said, and smiled to indicate I was kidding.

"He don't like anyone," Reggie said, and continued sipping a second beer that Lisa must have given him while I was rifling through my bag.

I excused myself to call Dr. Kumar to get approval to admit Reggie. Thankfully, the neighbor was no longer on the porch.

"Hey, I'm driving so I can't look at anything, just so you know," Dr. Kumar answered the phone.

"No problem. This is pretty straightforward."

I gave him the general rundown on Reggie. When I told him he had ascites, Dr. Kumar cut me off. "How bad?"

I scrolled to that part of the chart before realizing that I had gotten distracted talking to Reggie and Lisa and forgot to measure his stomach. My cheeks felt hot. "I'm so sorry, I forgot to measure. I'll go do it right now and call you back."

Dr. Kumar cut me off. "Hadley, I know you're a good nurse. It's okay. We're a team. Describe it to me."

I started to speak, but my mind went blank and I panicked because I could not think of any medical or professional way to describe what Reggie's stomach looked like. "I . . . I don't know. I really can get that measurement and call you back in two minutes."

"Does he look pregnant?" Dr. Kumar asked. That was exactly what I was thinking, but hadn't wanted to say.

"Yes, about nine months pregnant."

"He probably doesn't have much longer, with those lab results and that assessment. Admit him and send my condolences," Dr. Kumar said.

I agreed and hung up before taking a deep breath and stepping back inside Reggie and Lisa's home.

"Our physician gave me the okay to admit," I told the couple. As if he understood me, Max walked over to Reggie and placed his head on his owner's lap.

"Cheers to dying," Reggie said and chugged the remainder of his beer.

ON SATURDAY, I WOKE up to the sun coming through the window. I checked my phone and saw that Kelly had texted me to ask if I wanted to get my nails done. I'd had a rough week at work and all I felt like doing was lying on the couch and catching up on reality TV. The manufactured drama always made me forget about everything else going on in my life. "Not today, but next time for sure!" I texted back. I had about eight hours to decompress before another friend's birthday party, after which we were going to dinner at Chris's parents' house.

After watching a few shows and wrapping my friend's birthday gift, I got ready for the night. Despite the fact that it was still cold outside, I threw on jeans and a pink tank top—Chris's parents kept their house warm (but even then, Babette always seemed to be shivering now). I pulled my arm through my old fuzzy gray sweater and looked in the mirror. Not my best look, but it would do.

Chris was quick to compliment me when he walked in the room, telling me I looked beautiful. He looked nicer than usual, but he always made an effort when we were going to see my friends, which I appreciated.

We went to the party for an hour or so before saying our goodbyes and heading toward his parents' house. Once we pulled up, Chris pulled out his phone and said, "Oh, dang, they still aren't home from the grocery store." He gestured to the community dock outside of his parents' condo. "Want to walk out there for a minute?"

"Sure!" I agreed. The sun was just about to set, so our timing was perfect.

Hand in hand, we walked out to the dock, where a beautiful sailboat was tied to a post, bobbing in the water. Chris led me onto the boat.

"We can't do that," I whispered to him, laughing.

He turned back to me and smiled as I heard the captain say, "Welcome, Chris and Hadley!"

We cruised around the bay for a bit before docking at one of our favorite secluded beaches. Suddenly, it dawned on me why Kelly had invited me to get a manicure that morning. I grinned from ear to ear, savoring each second as I waited for the moment to happen.

We left the boat and walked on the sand until we reached the rocks. As we climbed onto them as we'd done so many times before, Chris got down on one knee. "Hadley, I would be honored to spend the rest of my life with you and Brody. Will you marry me?" he asked, smiling up at me.

"Yes!" I proclaimed without hesitation. After taking it all in, we headed back to the boat. The sun was long gone, but I was still able to make out the twinkle in Chris's eye that let me know the night wasn't over.

"One more surprise," he said, squeezing my hand. We docked at Louisiana Lagniappe, a waterfront restaurant, and said our goodbyes to the captain. Dinner wasn't the surprise, though.

"*Congratulations!*" I heard multiple voices cry out as we walked through the doors. As I scanned the room, I realized that all of our family and friends were there. My mouth hung open as I hugged everyone, but I was the most shocked to see my mom.

"*What?* I just talked to you! You were in Texas! You knew?" I asked her.

"I lied," my mom said through her tears. "Chris has been planning this for a long time. I'm so happy for you two."

I moved over to Babette, who admired my ring and told me how happy she was for us. "I know it's early, but do you have any dates in mind yet?" she asked.

I shrugged. "I mean, I've dreamed about my wedding day my whole life. I'll probably want to spend a long time planning. Maybe sometime next year," I said without thinking about Babette's own timeline.

"That sounds absolutely wonderful," Babette replied genuinely.

A moment later, I felt Chris's hand on my shoulder. He handed me a glass of champagne and we listened as a few people gave speeches and well-wishes for our future, including his parents. Each speech finished with all of our loved ones raising their glasses and exclaiming, "Cheers!"

ON MONDAY MORNING I was exhausted but happy, still riding high from the unexpected weekend festivities. I poured myself some coffee while listening to the morning meeting on speakerphone. As my co-workers gave their updates, I leaned on my kitchen countertop and admired the sparkling new ring on my left ring finger. I never wore jewelry, but I was excited to get used to wearing this.

"I saw Reggie a lot," Jenna, the weekend nurse, was saying. My ears perked up—time to pay attention. "He's having a rough time. Lots of pain and some confusion. His wife is not handling it well. She wants him to be a full code." I grimaced. A "full code" meant that if Reggie were to stop breathing, rather than calling time of death, we were instead mandated to call 911 and administer CPR. This was despite the fact that both Reggie and Lisa had already signed paperwork during admission and agreed to a do-not-resuscitate. Still, it sounded like Lisa didn't want that anymore. I made a mental note to see them first thing this morning.

WHEN I ARRIVED AT Reggie's home, the neighbor was out on his porch again. I smiled and waved.

"Is Reggie gonna die?" the neighbor yelled to me.

As badly as I wanted to pretend like I didn't hear him, it wasn't possible. "I can't share anything medical. It's against the law," I replied.

"I do a lot of things against the law," he countered. "Never got caught."

"Well, I have a baby at home so I need to stay employed and out of jail." I don't know why I was being so honest with a stranger—or even continuing the conversation at all, for that matter. "Have a good day," I said and knocked on Reggie's door.

This time Lisa didn't look as put together as she had when I last saw her. Max ran out from behind her and sped past me. "Get hit by a car for all I care!" Lisa yelled after him. I could tell she was at the end of her rope.

"Max! Treats!" I called. And with that magic word, he came bounding up the stairs and wagged his tail as he waited for his reward. I patted his head and pulled out my uneaten breakfast bar. Before handing it over, I looked at Lisa to make sure I could give it to him. She nodded her approval.

"Thank you," she said before bursting into tears. I quickly shut the door so Max couldn't run out again.

"I heard it was a rough weekend. We have options."

"The other nurse told me, and my answer is still no. No to the nursing home, no to the volunteer, no to the dying. I am not ready," she protested.

"Okay, how about this option?" I replied. "Go take a shower, get ready, and I will stay here and assess Reggie. Take your time."

"Okay," she said, relaxing. "Okay." She headed back toward the bedroom and I turned my attention to Max, who was lying on the ground near Reggie's recliner.

"Be a good boy for Momma, okay?" I said to Max. Max looked up at Reggie as if he wanted his opinion, but Reggie was fast asleep. I heard the shower turn on and lightly touched Reggie's arm to wake him. When that didn't work, I tried to say his name gently. I didn't want to startle him, but when I tried to gently shake him, Max barked loudly at me, rousing Reggie out of his slumber.

"Wha—what's going on?" Reggie startled.

"Hey! It's Hadley!"

"Oh, yeah I know you," he said, relaxing back into his chair.

"Can I ask you some questions?"

"Yeah, shoot," he replied, his eyes now closed again.

Reggie seemed okay to me, but I was still required to ask questions to determine if he was confused or not.

"Can you tell me your name?"

"That's a stupid question. Next one," he said. That wasn't an unusual answer to get so I decided to move on to the next question, and come back to this later.

"Can you tell me where you are right now?"

"Yeah, Mexia, Texas."

I looked up from my tablet to see if Reggie was joking, but he didn't appear to be. We were definitely not in Mexia, or anywhere even close to Texas.

"Can you tell me what year it is?"

"1977," he replied as if that was the obvious answer. "My grandmother said I need to hurry up."

"Really? Where are you going?"

"I don't know. Grandma is one of those people who you just listen to and don't ask questions," he replied.

"That makes sense. Did you see her or did she call you?"

"What a weird question. She's right there," he said, hitching his thumb to the left side of his chair. "Anything else or can I go back to sleep?"

"I think that's all of my questions," I said. I finished my assessment and shut down my tablet just as Lisa walked back into the room, looking refreshed. I smiled at her and asked if we could talk somewhere else so Reggie could sleep. She said yes and led me onto a covered back porch where we could still keep an eye on Reggie.

"So, he's seeing his deceased grandmother."

"Yes, and his parents," she said, lighting a cigarette and offering me one. I declined.

"What are your thoughts on that?"

"The doctors told us that he might get confused," she said, taking a long drag on the cigarette.

"So, I want you to know that I hate these conversations as much as you do. Seeing deceased loved ones and/or increased confusion are both signs that he is getting worse." I paused before continuing, speaking as gently as possible. "I heard that you want us to resuscitate him when he dies. We can do that, but I want to make sure that's what you really want."

Lisa sighed and wouldn't make eye contact with me as she took another drag from her cigarette. "I don't want my husband to die," she said.

"I get that." I paused and pondered how to handle the rest of this conversation. I thought back to my talk with Steve. "If he did pass soon, what would you consider to be a good death?" I asked.

This time, Lisa looked me directly in the eye and answered, "I don't know. Holding his hand. Telling him I love him."

"I completely agree," I said. "I want you to know that if he is a full code I will have to call 911 and start chest compressions immediately. The ambulance will take him to the hospital and the chances that he will walk out of that hospital are slim. They are not zero, but they're not good."

"Oh," Lisa replied quietly.

I glanced at Reggie through the glass window; he was still fast asleep with Max by his side. "You don't have to make the decision right now, but maybe it's a good thing to think about. I'm here to help you, but I don't want to overstep."

"I'm not used to making choices. I don't think I've ever made a decision in my life. Reggie and I have been together since we were teens, and he always made all the decisions. Then he got sick and we were shuffled around like cattle; test here, doctor's visit there, go see another specialist over in that town."

I nodded as Lisa spoke. It sounded very similar to Babette's situation. Lisa didn't know how much I truly understood her.

"Well, sleep on it," I advised.

Lisa nodded and we went back inside. I said my goodbyes to Reggie, who slept through the interaction, and gave Max a head scratch before heading out.

AROUND 7:00 P.M. I was stirring spaghetti sauce when I got a call. I placed the spoon down and answered the phone.

"Hello, this is the on-call nurse."

"Hi, this is Reggie's wife, Lisa. Um, I think he's going to die."

I shifted the phone to my other hand and said, "Hey, Lisa. It's Hadley. I'll be there soon."

"Oh, thank goodness," she said. I could hear the relief in her voice.

I hung up and was out the door within five minutes, shouting cooking instructions at Chris as I went.

A little more than a half hour later, I arrived at Reggie's home for the second time that day. I cautiously made my way through the grass, extra fearful of stepping into an unforeseen hole. The door was ajar so I peeked my head in while knocking. I looked around and didn't see anyone in the living room.

"Lisa? It's Hadley," I called out. Lisa appeared from around the corner and ushered me down a hallway to their bedroom, where Reggie was lying in bed. His breathing was loud and noisy. Max lay in the bed with him and whined.

"Has he had morphine?" I asked.

"Yes, just a few minutes ago. I've been giving it to him every few hours."

"You are doing such an amazing job," I assured her. "What

would he want us to do to make him comfortable? Some people like prayer, some like incense or candles, some like music."

"Um, he thinks everything goes black when you die, so no
prayer. I don't think we have any candles."

"What about music?" I asked.

"Country," she replied and looked at her husband lovingly.
"He likes country." She adjusted the old alarm clock radio on
their dresser until the station was playing today's country hits.

"Lisa," I said, "it's close. Do you want me to do CPR when
he passes?"

She ignored me and held her husband's hand, singing
along to the radio. I watched as she brushed back his hair and
told him how much she loved him. My heart rate picked up
when I heard his breathing slow, knowing it would soon stop
yet still not knowing what Lisa wanted me to do when that
moment arrived. If she wanted him to be resuscitated, then I
would have to start CPR immediately.

"If there's an afterlife, will you send me a sign, baby?" she
said to him. I watched as he took one more shallow breath.
Sometimes you're not sure if someone's breath will be their
last, but other times you just *know* it is. I knew it was Reggie's
last.

"Lisa," I said cautiously.

"No. Don't do anything," she said, continuing to hold his
hand. I didn't move.

At that moment, the radio host announced that "a special
request just came in for a special someone" and the crow of a
country singer soon followed.

"Randy Travis," Lisa said. "This was the song we danced to
at our wedding."

Chills ran up and down my spine.

"'Forever After All.' He picked it for our first dance." Lisa paused for several seconds. "How does forever work when one person is dead?" she asked, wiping her nose with her sleeve and standing up. "You can have them come get him. I'll be on the porch."

I was shocked by her response. Once she left the room, I went through my usual routine, including listening for a heartbeat, cleaning him up, and calling the funeral home. Max laid his head on Reggie's lap all the while.

Soon, there came the knock on the door. I greeted the funeral home workers, Dave and his partner, Sam, whom I recognized from previous deaths. Lisa came in when she heard them arrive and followed us into the bedroom. She was expressionless, completely devoid of emotion.

After preparing their gurney, Dave went to move Reggie over, but quickly stepped back when Max pounced onto Reggie's body and began growling aggressively. I had never seen Max growl. It was as if he knew.

"Max!" Lisa yelled before grabbing him by the collar and taking him out of the room. Dave and his co-worker transferred Reggie and covered him with a sheet before wheeling him out of the house. I walked back into the bedroom to check the sheets. Sometimes when patients are moved, they leave behind stains that can be disturbing, so I always throw the sheets into the wash before leaving. Max was already back on the bed, panting and whining as if he was crying. The sheets looked clean, so instead of doing the wash I tried to calm Max down by petting his head, but to no avail. After a few minutes, I went to look for Lisa to say my goodbyes.

She was on the back porch, smoking a cigarette. I went outside and closed the door behind me, unsure what to do or say.

"I never liked drinking," Lisa said. "But every time there was a promotion, or a wedding, or any other event, we felt like we needed to drink."

I sat down to show that I was listening and in no hurry.

"We had a lot to celebrate, I guess."

"That sounds like a good thing," I said tentatively.

"It was, but it led to a real problem. And now that very real problem has led to me being alone in my fifties. I have never been alone. What do I even do?" she asked. I didn't know how to answer that question.

"Well, we have a weekly support group," I tried. I watched as the trees in the field beyond us swayed slightly in the breeze.

Lisa smiled at me wanly in response. "You're sweet. Don't mess up your life like we did," she said, flicking the cigarette.

"I really enjoyed caring for Reggie. You did a great job caring for him. I mean that."

Lisa smiled and replied, "Thanks. I think this is goodbye now."

"Well, I think it's see you later," I tried again. I let her know that Steve offered weekly grief support meetings, and would also personally follow up with her throughout the next year.

"Thanks for everything, Hadley. Goodbye."

I took the hint and gathered my things, waving goodbye and giving Max a pat on the head as I left.

———

AFTER THE FORTY-MINUTE DRIVE home, I crawled into bed, exhausted. I felt uneasy about how things had ended with Lisa. I reached for my phone to text her, which is not explicitly against the rules, but also not something that we normally do.

"Thinking of you. I will call tomorrow," I typed and then pressed send. I watched as the DELIVERED status popped up on the screen, then put my phone down to charge before going to sleep.

When I woke up the next morning, I checked my phone and saw no response, so I went into the living room where Brody was happily playing with his trucks on the floor while Chris sipped coffee.

"Hey, I was thinking: Do you want to ask Steve to officiate our wedding?" Chris asked. I had already looked up officiants online, but no one stood out to me. I loved the idea of someone who had individual relationships with each of us officiating our wedding. "I love that!" I said, leaning down to kiss Brody on the top of his head. "I'll ask him at our meeting this morning."

I WAS THE FIRST to arrive at our weekly update meeting, where all departments come together to go through the status of each patient. Soon after I sat down, Steve rounded the corner and gave me a warm "Hello!"

Just the person I wanted to see. "Hi!" I chirped. "So, Chris and I were talking, and we'd be honored if you would officiate our wedding. Is that something you'd be up for?"

"I would be more than honored." He smiled at me.

I mouthed *Thank you* as more staff members filed into the room. We spoke about our patients in alphabetical order, which meant I was up first. In the middle of my spiel, our receptionist interrupted the meeting—something she had never done before.

"Travis," she said, holding her pinky and thumb up to her ear and mouth, indicating he had a phone call, "it's urgent." Travis walked out of the room and I continued speaking.

When Travis returned, he put his hand on Steve's shoulder and motioned for him to exit the room. I was confused, but tried to stay focused on a co-worker who was discussing a rapidly declining patient whose family needed more support.

Travis and Steve were gone while we continued with updates on two or three more patients, until Steve finally walked back in and said, "I'm so sorry to interrupt, but Hadley, we need you." Everyone looked at me as I stood up. I stepped outside and closed the heavy conference room door behind me, unsure what to expect.

"Hadley," Steve said, "it's about Reggie." I instantly replayed last night in my mind, wondering what could have possibly gone wrong. I couldn't think of anything. Reggie's death was calm, his wife didn't ask for CPR, and I watched the funeral home take him. I had even completed my charting and submitted it last night.

"Did you know his wife, Lisa?" Steve asked me.

Uh-oh, I thought. *This is because I texted her.* Maybe that wasn't okay to do after all.

"Yes, I texted her just so she would know someone cared about her," I explained.

Travis and Steve looked at each other, clearly confused,

and then Steve turned back to me. "Hadley, Lisa killed herself last night. The police think she did it right after you left."

I let his words sink in, but I didn't believe them. I could feel both of their eyes on me, but all I could do was shake my head in disbelief. After about a minute, I looked at Steve and said, "I should have known. I should have done something. This is my fault."

"Did she say she was suicidal?" Travis asked.

"No, but I was the last one to see her. I should have known, right?" I asked frantically.

Steve gave Travis a look to indicate he would handle it. He put his hand on my shoulder and told Travis, "We'll be back. Have another nurse take her patients today."

As soon as Travis was gone, I turned to Steve. "I need to go by their house. She isn't dead. He's wrong," I pleaded.

Steve sighed in response. "I have a better idea," he said. "Let's go somewhere else."

Feeling defeated, I nodded and followed him out to his car. After driving for about ten minutes, we turned down an old dirt road and I recognized where we were headed. Steve parked the car and turned off the engine. "Shall we?" he asked.

I was confused about why we were here, but I agreed. There wasn't a cloud in the sky, and the dust kicked up around my white sneakers as we walked. I was careful not to step on anyone's grave. Steve led me to a cement bench under a shady tree and we sat down. I knew exactly where we were, and I didn't want to look at the headstone. I didn't feel worthy of being at Carl's and Anna's graves today.

After a few moments, Steve said, "I met Carl's wife out here the other day to pray."

I looked at him. I didn't know they kept in touch.

"As I was looking around," he continued, "I noticed something that I think you should see too. Look around at the headstones."

I scanned the cemetery; so many last names of patients I had cared for stared back at me. "That's a lot of people I love," I said, tearing up.

"It's a whole lot, Hadley," he said. "It's a lot of peaceful passings you assisted with. It's also a heavy burden to carry, and I think it might be time to talk to a therapist. Not because anything is wrong with you, but because you're a good nurse and I don't want to see you burn out."

"I feel like the worst nurse ever today," I told him.

Steve put his arm around me and squeezed. "I know, kid. But better days are coming, okay?"

"We'll see," I replied.

Lily

I DIDN'T WANT TO NEED HELP. I WANTED TO BE ABLE TO disconnect and feel nothing. I wanted to be the star fiancée who held Chris's hand and comforted him through Babette's sickness, the doting mother who made Pinterest-worthy snacks for Brody's class, the world's best friend who remembered and coordinated everyone's birthday celebrations, and a full-time working nurse who handled all of her patients with the skill and ease of a Cirque du Soleil juggler.

At my first session with the therapist Steve recommended—a few weeks after Reggie's and Lisa's deaths—I tried to paint this picture of myself. But she wasn't buying it—and that made me uncomfortable. I had planned on seeing her for a session or two to work through the specific scenario that had led me here, but it was immediately clear that she had other ideas.

She began our first session with "How is your relationship with your parents?"

"My mom is great, but she lives in Texas now so I don't see

her much. My dad . . ." I trailed off and looked out the window at a bluebird on the tree right outside, briefly thinking about Mr. Carl. "It's complicated," I continued. "My parents divorced when I was seventeen, and then my dad and I spent years not speaking before we reconciled. Still, I wish my childhood was different."

"In what way?" the therapist asked.

How can you sum up a childhood? There were good parts and there were horrible parts, which I assumed was true for most people. I shrugged.

"My parents should have divorced much sooner. Their fights were really bad. But lots of people get divorced, it's normal."

"If you could rate your parents' fights on a scale of zero to ten with ten being the worst, what rating would you give them?"

"Ten," I replied immediately.

"That is not normal," she said, without taking her eyes off me. I squirmed in my seat. "On that note, how is your relationship with your fiancé?"

"Good! We have fights, too, of course, but he's a great guy. I finally don't feel like a single mom anymore. His mom is really sick, so we spend a lot of time with his family."

"And how do you feel about that?"

No part of me liked feeling this vulnerable. I wanted to run, but instead I sat still and tried to keep my composure. "It's tough," I replied honestly. "I love my fiancé, and I love his family. I'm grateful to them and how they've accepted my son and me. But it's difficult waiting for someone to die. It feels like we're putting our lives on hold, and that's stressful. But even thinking those thoughts makes me feel like a horrible person, compared to what Chris and his family are going through. And I love Babette too." I paused for a moment before continuing. "I'm a hospice nurse. I watch families care for and deal with losing loved ones all the time. I know it's hard and I know it's stressful and emotional for everyone involved. But it's still difficult when it's your own family."

The therapist nodded. "Do you and your fiancé fight because of this?"

I looked at her blankly.

"I'm going to assume that you never learned to fight," she said, scribbling something onto her notepad.

"I'm sorry?"

"You didn't have a healthy example of how to have a disagreement within a romantic relationship, right?"

I nodded in response. I hadn't expected our conversation to go in this direction.

"We can work on that. It's okay. I know that your work as a hospice nurse is why you came to see me, but I believe in treating the whole person, not just isolated parts."

I let out a sigh of relief. I felt better knowing she had a plan.

I FELT MORE RELAXED when I returned to the therapist's office for our next session.

"We're going to discuss the suicide today," she stated plainly.

All of my confidence disappeared. I gulped nervously and

reached for my water bottle. I still felt immense guilt about Lisa's death, no matter how much I tried to distract myself. It felt like an elephant was constantly sitting on my chest. Even though no one said any such thing to me, I felt like everyone in the office must think I was a horrible nurse for not preventing it.

"You said last week that you feel personally responsible," the therapist said.

I nodded. "If I would have stayed then I could have stopped her. I should have stayed."

The therapist leaned back in her chair, raised her eyebrows, and replied, "You think you have that power?"

I looked at her quizzically.

"You don't think she would have done it no matter how long you stayed?"

I let her words settle over me. She was probably right, but I still felt like there was something more I could have done.

"What indicators did you miss that would have prompted you to stay?" she asked.

"I don't know, but I'm sure there were some."

"Look, hindsight is always twenty-twenty." The therapist leaned in toward me, looking me directly in the eye. "If I gave you an indicator that I was going to do something to harm myself right now, would you leave?"

"Of course not!" I quickly responded.

"Then that tells me that you didn't have any idea she was going to do what she did. If you had, you would have stayed. You didn't do anything wrong, and I doubt she wants you to feel this way."

With those words, I felt something release inside me. The heavy weight I'd been carrying around was starting to lift. Maybe not the full elephant, but at least a foot or two.

"Now, let's talk about some other things," she said, and we moved on.

THE NEXT MORNING, I entered the office feeling a little lighter. "Hey!" I greeted Will, the eleventh-hour volunteer who had sat by Elizabeth's bed on Christmas. Every now and then he made an appearance in the office, usually for computer training or some other sort of administrative procedure.

"Well, hello there," he said. "I heard about Reggie and his wife. I'm so sorry." His kind eyes held mine as he spoke.

"Me too. I thought caring for patients my age or younger was the hardest part of the job, but that was awful."

Will nodded and we stood in silence for a few seconds, as if acknowledging the pain. After a moment he said, "I'm guessing I'll be seeing you more at night for a bit, huh?"

I looked at him, confused. Will raised his eyebrows when he realized I hadn't heard the news yet. "One on-call nurse is taking family leave to care for her new grandbaby, and the other one just turned in her notice," he informed me.

I groaned. I already worked every Monday through Friday from 8:00 A.M. to 5:00 P.M., picked up Brody from school, made dinner, put him to bed, then charted for a few hours before falling asleep myself—usually on the couch, utterly exhausted. At our last meeting, we were told that we might be able to hire another nurse soon, but for now it was just the three of us full-time nurses running around, trying to care for fifty patients between us. And now it sounded like the three of us would be rotating nights as well, with both of our night-time nurses out of the picture.

I hoped that Travis had a solution for the on-call nurses. Apparently, he did not.

"So, we will soon have no on-call nurses," Travis began our weekly meeting. We all looked at each other. I shifted uncomfortably in my chair. "We have advertised the jobs as being open, but there's no interest right now," he continued.

"So, it goes without saying that we will not be accepting new patients then, right?" Jenna asked, cutting him off mid-sentence.

"Well, not exactly," Travis replied. "Corporate would still like for us to keep accepting new patients and rotate on-call."

"Let me get this straight. You want us to continue working without lunch breaks every day, spend hours every night charting at home, and then not sleep every third night on top of that? I'm not entertaining this. I have patients to see and this meeting could have been an email," Jenna said before pushing herself back from the table, gathering her things, and leaving. Amanda and I looked at each other, shocked. I secretly wished I had Jenna's confidence, but there was no way I would ever question authority like that—at least not out loud.

"Let's take it night by night for right now," Travis said. "Hadley, I have you on for tonight."

I nodded. It didn't feel like I had a choice, and I knew our patients needed someone to care for them. As I walked out of the office right before 5:00 P.M., I called Chris to explain the situation and was grateful that he was willing to help with Brody.

"They better be paying you well, though," he said.

"Two dollars an hour." We were paid two dollars an hour to wait for the phone to ring, then our hourly rate in the event we did go out on a call. Although waiting for the phone to ring doesn't require much, your life is on hold in case it does, at which point you have to be ready to fly out the door at a moment's notice.

"Is that legal?" Chris asked, flabbergasted.

"You know I won't speak up and risk my job."

"You never sleep when you're on call. I don't like that you're going to be doing this so often."

"I know. It gives me a lot of anxiety," I admitted. "I always worry I won't hear my phone and I'll be fired." Although I couldn't see Chris, it was almost like his concern somehow transferred itself through the phone, despite his silence. "I'll be okay though!" I said quickly, trying to stay optimistic. "I mean, it's not like I have a choice."

WHEN I GOT HOME, I felt my anxiety creeping in as I checked my phone for the millionth time, making sure I hadn't missed a call. My phone stayed silent as I made dinner and gave Brody a bath. It continued to stay silent as I charted while Chris watched the news beside me on the couch.

"Have you thought about how many bridesmaids you'll have?" Chris asked.

"Well, I know I'll have at least the five friends that I regularly talk to, with Summer as my maid of honor. What about you?"

"I want to have six. What about Hannah? You always speak so fondly of her."

It's true that Hannah was one of my oldest and dearest friends. We'd been through so much together. But she'd moved out of state a few years ago, and in the chaos of life, we didn't have a chance to catch up very often. At this point, I felt out of the loop with her life. "I haven't spoken to her much since she moved," I replied.

"Yeah, but y'all have been through a lot together. You should consider it."

I shrugged. "We don't talk much anymore."

I checked my phone again. Nothing. As I continued charting, my mind kept wandering to Hannah and asking her to be my bridesmaid. We had been friends since we were fourteen, and the loss of Taylor Haugen had bonded us in high school. But it was the time she had spent with me when I was pregnant with Brody that Chris was referring to, that I spoke of so fondly. When many of my friends distanced themselves, she leaned in. She called to check in on me every day. She worked overtime to help me buy baby clothes even though I insisted that I didn't need them. She helped my mom throw my baby shower, and I had an inkling that she made sure everyone showed up to support me.

She had moved to North Carolina with her longtime boyfriend, however, and we hadn't talked much since. I was busy, and, from what I could see on social media, she looked busy too. I couldn't help but feel jealous when I scrolled through her Instagram feed and saw all the new friends she was making in North Carolina. It seemed like she'd moved on.

"I need to take a shower. Can you answer the phone if it rings?" I asked Chris, handing my phone to him.

"What do I say?" he asked.

"Just say hello and that I'm in the shower. It should be someone from the call center, just another nurse."

As I lathered up my hair under the warm water, I started to daydream about our wedding. After a few minutes, I finally felt my body relax, only to be interrupted by Chris opening the bathroom door and shouting at me that the phone was ringing.

I quickly turned off the water and grabbed the towel, wiping my hands so I could take the phone from him.

"Hello? I need help," I heard a voice say. It sounded like a young girl. Although the call center was supposed to be on the line as well, every now and then they transferred a patient call to us and hung up immediately, rather than staying on the line.

"Hi. Yes, I'm a registered nurse. What can I help with?"

"We're twenty minutes away. I need you to meet me there," she said before the line went dead. I stared at the phone, confused. I threw on my scrubs and called the phone number back, but it rang and rang without anyone picking up. I had no idea who needed me and I had no idea where I needed to go. I tried the on-call number and, thankfully, they were able to tell me which patient had called by tracing the phone number: Lily Webster. I scrolled through a long list of patients on my tablet and clicked on her name to read the last note from the nurse—but her chart was blank. I clicked over to my work email and searched her name there.

"Hey team, we have a patient that's traveling in from

Georgia. We will only have her for a few days. It was a last-minute trip, but the hospice company she's with in Georgia said she's stable and should not need a visit. I'll upload the documents to her chart tomorrow," an email from our receptionist read. So, Lily was a travel patient.

Because Destin is a tourist destination, we frequently receive travel patients. These are patients who have a hospice company in their hometown that asks us to be on call in case of an emergency. These patients usually don't call us because people who are very sick usually don't feel up to traveling. There's also the fact that some state laws can make interstate travel difficult should a patient die, which can deter some hospice patients from traveling—although, unfortunately, many aren't aware of these laws until it's too late.

When these traveling patients *do* call, it can be tricky because we usually don't have a lot of information about them, and they're only going to call us if there's a crisis. Lily, apparently, was a patient in crisis, and I was going into this visit blind. I hopped into my car and put the address into my GPS system. I drove up to a condo on the beach and parked next to the community pool, then pulled out my tablet to see what unit I was going to. "3B, 3B, don't forget that," I said to myself as I walked into the building. The walkways to the unit were outside and the wind was coming from the north, fierce and cold.

"Come in!" I heard someone yell when I knocked on the door. I let myself in, and the scent of cleaning chemicals instantly hit me. Past the short entryway was a large U-shaped kitchen, where two black suitcases sat by the door, still packed. I could see my reflection in the floor-to-ceiling windows that lined the wall, which I'm sure gave way to a spectacular view of the ocean during the day. But right now, it only mirrored the chaos in front of me. A young woman in her early twenties was pacing back and forth, clearly frantic. Another young woman, who I assumed was Lily, was sitting on the couch with her head thrown back against the cushion, her arms limp by her sides. She wore a crocheted pink and brown hat, which I guessed was covering a bald head. She was pale and motionless.

"Hi, I'm the nurse," I said, moving toward Lily.

"She was fine," her friend told me pleadingly. "She asked me to take her to the beach one last time. We got in the car. We were singing. We got snacks. She took a nap and about half an hour before we arrived I looked over at her and she looked like this."

I nodded in response. Travel often took more out of hospice patients than either the patient or their traveling companion might expect.

"It kinda scared me, but I told Lily we were almost there and to wake up. She didn't move. So I said it louder. Nothing. Then I started yelling. Nothing. When we got here, I parked and ran over to her side of the car. I opened the door and she practically fell out of the car, like a sack of potatoes. I had to carry her inside. Like a baby." The girl's eyes were red from crying and mascara had stained her face.

"What's your name?" I asked gently.

"Allison," she said, her voice catching.

"Okay, Allison. Let me assess Lily quickly. Then we can come up with a plan, okay?" Allison nodded, but didn't stop pacing while I took Lily's vital signs.

The first thing I noticed was that her breathing was labored. "Does she have any medications?" I asked. Allison left the room to grab them and was back in under a minute. I rifled through the box until I found the bottle labeled ROXANOL, a brand name for morphine. It was full. "Has she taken any?" I asked, assuming the answer was no.

"No," Allison confirmed.

I read the side of the bottle, which instructed that she take the lowest dose, 0.25 mL. "Does she have any allergies?"

"I have no idea. We were just supposed to go to the beach!" Allison replied anxiously.

"Okay, it's okay," I said calmly. I pressed on the sides of the dropper and pulled up 0.25 mL into the syringe. I placed the tip of the dropper inside Lily's cheek and pressed the sides of the dropper again to release the medicine into Lily's mouth. It would be absorbed into her cheek and she would not need to swallow it, thankfully.

"Is that going to kill her?"

"No, it's going to help her breathing—but she may not have much longer."

Allison stopped pacing immediately and stared straight ahead before looking at Lily. After staring in silence for a moment, she suddenly ran into the kitchen and began rifling through the drawers. I had no idea how to react or what to say as I knelt by Lily and observed her, making sure she didn't have an adverse reaction to the medicine. Not even a minute later, Allison practically sprinted out the front door.

Maybe she needs a minute to herself. That had to have been rough to hear, I thought. I turned back to Lily and watched her chest rise and fall. Her breathing was still labored and ragged, and her lips were almost as white as her skin. She was my age, I realized. I wondered what had led her to this moment. How long ago had she found out that she was dying? I wondered about everything she had been through that finally led up to the decision to go into hospice.

It was time to assess her heart rate. Instead of using my stethoscope, I decided to take her pulse via her wrist. I grabbed Lily's hand and turned it over. She had a semicolon tattoo, which caught me off guard; these tattoos are commonly a symbol for an unsuccessful suicide attempt. I wondered if Lily had gotten it before or after her diagnosis, and thought about how tragic it would be if she had survived an attempted suicide only to end up here.

I waited for the hand on my watch to reach the twelve so I could begin counting. After just the first ten seconds, it was already clear that her heart rate was not as strong, steady, or fast as normal. I continued counting, but was interrupted by the front door opening again. I looked over and saw Allison barreling toward us with a bowl of sand in her hands. Confused and a little scared, I dropped Lily's wrist and moved out of the way.

I watched in awe as Allison leaned over and placed the bowl of sand on the ground near Lily. She then moved past me and threw open all the sliding glass doors that I now saw led out to a large balcony. The sticky, salty air immediately blew into the condo, and the silence that had permeated the room was replaced by the howling of the wind and crashing of waves. Allison knelt in front of Lily as if she was praying. With fresh tears streaming down her face, she removed Lily's bright green sneakers one at a time, then grabbed the bowl of sand and placed Lily's bare feet into it. Allison lovingly grabbed Lily's hand and stroked her fingers, repeating over and over, "You made it, Lil. You made it to the beach. I love you. You made it." I watched as one tear fell down Lily's cheek and onto her T-shirt. Allison cried harder.

Then, as if the universe knew, the wind stopped along with Lily's breath. All was silent for a moment before Allison's sobs filled the room.

AS I WALKED OUT of the condo, I thought about my own friends. Who would do that for me? And who would I be that person for? The answer was obvious to me, and I suddenly understood that no amount of time or geography was ever going to change that. I pulled out my phone with one person in mind. "Hi! I have a question for you," I texted. "When I say 'I do,' I want people by my side who have *always* been by my side. Even if we don't talk every day, I know you'd drop anything for me. Will you be my bridesmaid?"

The reply from Hannah popped up on my phone before I had even made it back to my car: "Of course! I love you forever!!"

I smiled and put my phone back in my bag, a sense of calm overtaking me.

Babette

NOW THAT I HAD MY BRIDESMAIDS SETTLED, CHRIS and I started discussing potential wedding dates one February night. Living in Florida, we both knew that the stifling summer months were out.

"Pretty much every Saturday in the fall is out too. I don't want people trying to watch football while we're walking down the aisle," Chris said, only half joking.

"I've never imagined getting married in the winter."

"I guess that leaves next spring then," he said, looking at the calendar.

"A spring wedding sounds great!" I could imagine it already: pastel colors, warm but not too-hot weather, refreshing drinks, and that last feeling of calm right before too many tourists showed up for the summer months. "Next spring it is! Let's go through our must-haves and nice-to-haves next," I told him as I brought up the wedding planning template I'd found on Google. The two of us hunched over the computer.

"Setting—maybe the beach?" Chris suggested.

"Yes, but maybe *near* the beach, not on it. I kinda hate the idea of a long dress and sand."

"Agreed." He nodded. We continued to scroll.

"Live band or DJ?" Chris read.

"I'm not picky," I said.

"Me neither," he echoed, as he kept scrolling. And then, suddenly, he stopped. I scanned the page and saw the wedding planning step that had caught his attention: *Choose a song for the mother-son dance.* I felt sick to my stomach. Next spring was more than a year away. Although we sat in silence, both of us were thinking the same thing: Babette wouldn't be here next spring.

Chris quietly closed the laptop and walked away. Once I heard him start up the lawnmower, a task that probably didn't need to be done but would help him clear his mind, I re-opened the computer and searched for the most popular mother-son wedding songs. A YouTube playlist popped up. I pressed play on the first song on the list, closed my eyes, and listened. What would our wedding look like without Babette? One less parent to walk Chris down the aisle. An empty seat in the front row. No mother-son dance. Family pictures with a gaping hole where Babette should have been.

I had always assumed that it took a year or more to plan a wedding—it had for all of my friends, at least. But was that *really* necessary? Was there any reason Chris and I couldn't plan a wedding in the next couple of months? I imagined what our wedding would be like if I didn't spend a year plan-ning it. I might not get my first-choice wedding venue. Some people might not be able to make it. I might not be able to find my dream dress. But none of those things even came close to the sadness we would all feel if Babette wasn't there on our wedding day. The answer was obvious.

I walked outside and found Chris staring at nothing, clearly deep in thought.

"What about this May?" I asked him.

"Like, in three months?"

"Yeah, why not?" I looked at him, shielding my eyes from the sun. I could feel the big smile stretching across my face.

Chris smiled back at me and gave me a big hug. "Thank you," he said.

I felt so much happiness in that moment. There was no doubt that I had made the right choice.

THE UNIVERSE SEEMED TO have my back, and everything for the wedding began to fall into place. I found a venue with a beautiful rooftop that overlooked the beach. They had never hosted a wedding before but had been wanting to start, so they agreed to give us a substantial discount in exchange for using our wedding photos on their website. I went wedding dress shopping with my mom, expecting to have to pay a ton of money for rush shipping, but the dress I loved happened to be one I could take home that same day. Although a few friends couldn't attend, most people could—including all of our bridesmaids and groomsmen. I wasn't picky when it came to choosing vendors; I went with whoever was available, and they were all outstanding.

Babette never imposed on our wedding planning, and only offered advice when asked. I gave her the task of choosing her dress in whichever color she preferred, and the song for the mother-son dance. When she went dress shopping she sent me pictures of the contenders, asking my preference. Even the extra-small dresses seemed to swallow her up. I told her they were all beautiful.

IN THE NEXT FEW MONTHS, Babette stopped wanting to do much that required leaving the house. She was nauseous due to the chemotherapy and was losing even more weight. When Chris and I went out to dinner with Babette and Tom, she often pushed her food away. I could see the pain behind Chris's eyes every time this happened.

"You have to eat, Mom," he begged her one night.

She immediately changed the subject. "I picked out our song. I want our dance to be to 'Good Riddance' by Green Day."

I didn't say anything, but I wondered if Babette was confused. That was definitely not a song I had seen on any of the top mother-son dance song lists, nor had I ever heard her mention Green Day before.

Back in our car after dinner, I searched for the song on Spotify and pressed play. Chris and I sat there crying as we listened to Green Day sing about the unpredictability of life and how everything happens for a reason. *I hope you had the time of your life.*

A few months later, I watched Chris and Babette dance to the song at our wedding. It was perfect. As the tears fell freely, I silently thanked my makeup artist for having the foresight to choose waterproof mascara. When the song ended, I felt a hand on my back and turned to find Steve. I hugged him through my tears, and he hugged Chris with his other arm when he walked off the dance floor.

"Proud of you two," he said before giving Babette a hug too. It was a magical night.

MANY PEOPLE WHO HAVE a loved one with a terminal illness find themselves either altering their plans because of it or putting life on hold. Death is like birth: You know it's coming, but the timing is unpredictable (only even more so in the case of death), and it's an anxiety-ridden process of waiting. While we wanted to go to Greece for our honeymoon, Chris and I ultimately decided we didn't feel comfortable being that far away, just in case.

That summer, Babette didn't spend her days on the beach as she usually did. She slept much more and ate even less than she had been. We rarely went out, choosing instead to eat dinner with Chris's parents at their house. As the summer turned into fall, Babette's confusion started to become evident and her scans didn't look promising. I wondered if it was time for hospice, but I didn't want to be the one to suggest it.

Chris's brother Nick took leave from work and came from Louisiana to help. When he had to return after a few months, Tom, Chris, and I rotated taking time off to take Babette to doctors' appointments or stay at the house with her to help her go to the bathroom and make sure she didn't fall, on the rare occasions when she got out of bed. When she reached the point where she was barely able to form sentences and spent the vast majority of her day sleeping, the oncologist recommended hospice.

I knew Chris's family would turn to me for guidance, and I had already spent a lot of time weighing different options. Some days I thought it would be best to keep my personal and private life separate by choosing a company that I didn't work for. Other days, I felt like having Babette under my company's care would give me more control. Ultimately, I didn't trust anyone except for Dr. Kumar, the nurses in my company, and Steve to care for her. I called Travis to let him know that it was time, and he sent Amanda out to assess and admit Babette.

It was odd to be on the other side of the conversation I'd had with patients so many times before. Amanda did things in a different order than I did, which meant that I didn't know what part was coming next. My heart dropped when I saw the bright yellow DO NOT RESUSCITATE form and knew where we were headed. "So, if her heart stops naturally, signing this form means that we won't intervene," Amanda explained to Tom. She said this in the same tone she'd used to explain the insurance paperwork. *Did I do that? Did I act as if something as serious as a DNR was just another piece of paper to sign?* I hoped not, and swore I would never do so from this moment forward. Tom signed the form, and I was grateful I didn't have to convince him to do so.

Once Babette was on hospice, one of my co-workers came by every day, but other than the thirty minutes or so that they were there, it was quiet. On the days when we weren't already with her during the day, Chris, Brody, and I went by every day after work. Brody was too young to really understand what was happening. I spent most of those days feeling like I should seize the moment, like I should be doing *something* instead of just sitting there with her, but I wasn't sure what to do. Most of the time, we just told Babette how much we loved her.

We think of death and dying as being so gray and serious—and, of course, in many ways it is. But amidst that, there are also moments of levity and humor, even if that humor is sometimes dark. One day, Chris asked me if I thought Holly would be waiting to greet his mom on the other side.

In the early days of our relationship, Chris had come off the field from a kickball game only to find a phone screen full of missed calls. "I missed ten calls from my brother and Dad," he told me, looking alarmed. Although neither of us said it, both of us were sure something had happened to Babette.

Chris called his brother Eric as we jogged back to the car and learned that the calls were actually about the family's sixteen-year-old Western terrier, Holly, who had suddenly become sick. We rushed to Chris's parents' house, where we were greeted by complete chaos. Tom was at the dining room table and Eric was on the floor sitting next to Babette, who was cradling Holly in a blanket. Surveying the scene, Chris said, "We have to take her to the vet."

"If we take her to the vet, they're going to put her down," Babette said through tears. "We can't let them do that!"

We all looked at each other, unsure how to handle the situation. It somehow felt wrong to convince a person who was dying that the best thing for another creature was to die. Leaning down, Chris explained to his mom with as much sensitivity as possible how taking Holly to the vet was an act of kindness and the best thing for her. Finally, Babette agreed.

The vet tried everything he could, but after several hours it became clear that the time had come to let Holly go. At two o'clock that morning, we all gathered around Holly in a sterile veterinary room to say goodbye.

Once we got Holly's ashes back a few weeks later, Babette was adamant that the entire family schedule a time to spread them. But with four grown kids living in different states, that was easier said than done. Until the holidays rolled around, that is. Everyone was in town that Christmas and we had all gathered together over a huge lunch. Chris and I had a few hours before we were due to be at my dad's house, and I was looking forward to sneaking a nap in first. Just as I was about to figure out how to make a polite exit, Babette clapped her hands and said, "Come on! We're going to the beach."

"Right *now*? Can't we go later?" Chris's sister CJ asked.

"Right now. Come on!" Babette commanded, waving her arms as she spoke to emphasize that she meant right this second.

Obediently, we all got up and piled into our cars to go to the beach. As we walked along the boardwalk, we hugged our jackets tightly around ourselves in an attempt to block the strong wind that was blowing off the water. It was clear that, with the exception of Babette, no one wanted to be here.

Once we were on the beach, we all stood in the sand a few feet away from the water. Babette pulled out the large ziplock bag that held Holly's ashes and began walking down to the ocean. Although, in hindsight, what happened next should have been obvious, none of us saw it coming.

Babette opened the bag, grabbed a fistful of ashes, and threw them into the water. Except, thanks to the strong wind, the ashes didn't actually go into the water. Instead they did a quick airborne U-turn and flew back to the beach, scattering themselves over all of us.

"*Stop! Stop!*" we all cried out to Babette, who seemed oblivious to what was happening. She obliged for a moment, just long enough to call back to us: "We are doing this! I don't want to hear the negativity." With that, she continued to throw more large fistfuls of ashes into the wind. By the time she finished and walked back toward us, we were all in hysterics from the ducking and dodging we'd done as Holly's remains flew back at us. We tried to pull ourselves back together as Babette placed her hand on her heart and solemnly said, "Holly will always be in our hearts."

"Yeah, and in our lungs," Chris cracked, causing everyone to burst into uncontrollable laughter.

LITTLE DID I KNOW that the wind would have an impact on Babette's death too. For several weeks, her hospice experience went smoothly. She never suffered any pain or discomfort, and most of the time she just slept. And then came a factor completely out of our control. "Hurricane Michael expected to become a major hurricane," the breaking news headline blared. Chris and I watched as the weatherman pointed out the storm's potential landfall areas across the coast. Our home looked to be right in the middle of it. I groaned in frustration. Hurricanes are the absolute worst.

"It could do anything right now, so let's not freak out yet," Chris said before flipping the television to a different channel.

Less than twenty-four hours later, both our home and his parents' home were under mandatory evacuation orders. I went into Dr. Kumar's office to ask him what our options were. "Evacuating is going to be really tough with Babette," I told him. "I think it would be easier to stay here, but she is getting worse."

"Hadley, I'm going to be honest with you: When that hurricane hits they'll pull everyone off the roads, including EMS. You can call, but no one will come. I do not want you to be in a situation where you need assistance but can't get any," he told me flatly.

"So, we have to evacuate?" I asked.

Dr. Kumar nodded glumly.

NONE OF US WANTED to move Babette, but we didn't feel like we had any other option, so that's what we did. During hurricanes, healthcare facilities usually have an A-team that consists of people who hunker down for the storm. As soon as the roads open back up, the B-team relieves the A-team and works to resolve the chaos and fallout in the days that follow. Chris and I explained our situation and begged our employers to place us on the B-team so we could evacuate with Babette.

After getting approved for the B-team, we secured our home as best we could, putting up the hurricane shutters and bringing in anything that might fly away. Then we quickly packed up our car to evacuate to my mom and stepdad's rental home in Biloxi, Mississippi, a few hours away. I was a little nervous about going to Mississippi with Babette because of how difficult and expensive it can be to transfer someone back to their home state if they pass away out of state, but we had no choice.

Babette did well on the ride, summoning up the energy to sit upright in the passenger seat of her and Tom's car. Brody and I followed in another car, and Chris in a third, so that we could all return on our necessary timelines once the roads were open and the B-teams were called in.

For the next two days, all we did was watch the news and care for Babette. We tried to get her to eat, but even sips of water caused her to cough. When she wasn't sleeping, she stared at the television wordlessly. I wondered if she knew what was going on. Watching a storm is always such a helpless feeling, wondering if you'll have a home to come back to, wondering if your co-workers and patients are okay. And I think we all felt particularly helpless during this storm.

"The eye of the storm has made landfall in Mexico Beach as a Category Five hurricane," the reporter announced as the TV played in the background. We all turned to watch the update. The hurricane had hit further east than expected, which meant our homes would probably survive. Within the hour, Chris and I were contacted by our managers.

"They want me there by 8:00 A.M.," Chris said, hanging up with his boss.

"The storm hasn't even passed yet. I don't want you on the roads!" I protested.

"I'll leave at 5:00 A.M. I don't have a choice."

"I have an admission for you at 10:00 A.M.," Travis texted me shortly thereafter.

"Guess I'll be right behind you," I told Chris, showing him the text.

———

AS PLANNED, CHRIS LEFT in his scrubs early the next morning, planning to go straight to work. Two hours later, I did the same. Thankfully, Brody's daycare was open and I was able to drop him off on my way to the admission. Tom and Babette stayed behind.

Because of where the storm hit, I had assumed that there was minimal damage in our town, but I was wrong. I drove in to find tree limbs down everywhere and the entire town, except for emergency services and some daycares, still shuttered.

With Brody safely in daycare, I called Tom to check in on the way to see my patient. Babette was doing about the same: sleeping and barely eating. We decided that it would be best for him to head home with her so that she could be in a familiar environment. I promised that I would try to come by as soon as I was done with the admission.

My patient and his wife were both lovely, and all was going well until the time came to order his medications. The phone rang and rang when I dialed the number for their preferred pharmacy until, finally, an automatic message clicked on. *"We are currently closed due to Hurricane Michael and hope to open again soon."* I looked up the number to another pharmacy and tried again. Same message, different phrasing. Finally, after about thirty minutes of trying every pharmacy nearby, I called Travis.

"Travis, do you know any pharmacies that are open?" I asked him.

"You're not the only one with this issue. If you're calling just for billing purposes, we can handle that tomorrow. If they need medications, though, they need to go to the hospital," he told me.

"Oh, wow. My patient is okay. Anything else I should know, though?"

"If any of your patients need to go to the hospital then they can't go to our usual hospital. They have to go to Fort Walton Beach."

"What? That's a lot farther away! It could be over an hour drive for some of my patients!"

"Have you seen the news today?" he asked me. I hadn't because I had left so early in the morning. "Bay Medical Center is not okay. I don't even know how to describe the damage. Most of their patients were transported to our hospital. They have critical care patients in the hallways. Do not, under any circumstances, send any of our patients there."

"Okay, but my mother-in-law is not doing well. Once I finish up here, I really need to go help my father-in-law care for her."

"Last I heard she wasn't critical," Travis replied. "Your patients need you just as much as she does."

"I already left her this morning to come do this admission. Please," I begged, feeling close to tears. "What if I call to check on all my patients?"

"Okay. That's fine, but I need notes on all of them too."

I FINISHED UP MY admission and encouraged my new patient to call if he needed anything at all. Once we were done, I ran out the door to my car. I had about thirty minutes before Tom and Babette would be home to call all seventeen of my patients. About halfway through my calls, Tom called.

"We're getting close to home," he updated me, sounding calm enough, "but her breathing seems odd."

"Oh, that can happen," I assured him. "I'll be done in just a few minutes and will head your way so I can help." I figured we could treat Babette's labored breathing with medications we already had on hand or by positioning her differently. After I finished my calls, I put my car into reverse and backed down the long driveway to head toward my in-laws' home. As I drove, I observed the damage from the hurricane and had to swerve a few times to avoid debris.

As I pulled up to their condo, I saw Tom's car.

"Perfect timing!" I said. But when I saw Babette, I was shocked. She was gasping for air and practically unconscious. It seemed she had deteriorated rapidly over the course of the three-hour car ride.

"I need the bottle labeled Roxanol," I instructed Tom.

He went to the trunk to grab it. "I can't find the medication bag," he said, panicking.

And then it hit me. I felt lightheaded as I realized I had forgotten to put the medication back in the bag before I'd left this morning. "I—I'm so sorry," I stammered. "I put them in the refrigerator," I told him, tearing up. Her medication was best kept in the refrigerator, and since I was always the one giving Babette her meds, I hadn't thought to tell anyone else. Normally, I could call the pharmacy and get a new prescription, but I already knew there were no pharmacies to call.

"Okay, here's what we have to do," I told Tom. "We have to take her to the hospital for some medicine. Once we get it, we can come back home." It was clear to me from looking at her that Babette was now actively dying, which meant we had about seventy-two hours if she followed a typical timeline. Although it wouldn't be fun to take her to the hospital in this state, we had enough time to get Babette her medicine, bring her back home where she was comfortable, and make sure that all of the kids arrived in time to say their goodbyes.

I hopped into the backseat as Tom drove and Babette slumped over in the front, no longer able to hold herself up as she had on the car ride just three days earlier. The long drive to the hospital seemed even longer with each gasping breath Babette took. The one thing I was supposed to do was to keep her at home and comfortable, and I was failing. I debated whether or not I should call Chris at work. I didn't want him to leave if he didn't have to, and I felt confident that Babette had at least a few days left. But still, something told me that I should let him know. My hands shook as I picked up the phone.

"Hey, babe," I said when Chris answered, trying to keep my voice as calm as possible. "So, we have to go to the hospital for your mom. Um, I don't think you need to come, but I wanted to let you know. We have to go to Fort Walton Beach. I know that's far for you and I really don't think you need to come."

"Actually, they sent me to the Fort Walton Beach clinic today because of the hurricane. I'm just across the street from the hospital and most of my patients didn't show up today," he told me. "Call me when you get here."

———

AS WE ARRIVED AT the hospital, I told Tom to pull the car up to the ER entrance so I could get Babette into a wheelchair. Chris, who had been on the lookout, saw us and jogged over to help. He held his mother upright as we rolled her into the hospital, and I hurriedly explained the situation to the receptionist. She ran back to get a nurse who showed us to a bed in the hallway. A doctor came over immediately to order medications that would provide relief for Babette's agonal breathing. Everything was happening quickly, and it suddenly seemed clear that Babette was not going to make it back home. I couldn't believe it—after all of the patients who I'd been able to provide with a comfortable, peaceful passing, in the end I couldn't manage that for my own mother-in-law.

As the nurse administered the medications for Babette's breathing, Tom called the rest of the kids so they could say their goodbyes on speakerphone. I watched helplessly while Tom held the phone up by Babette's face as CJ and then Nick told her how much they loved her. Doctors, nurses, patients, and strangers walked by, looking at Babette as they passed. I felt like I was going to have a breakdown; *this was all so wrong!* I had spent years learning exactly what a good death looked like, and I had planned that for Babette. There would be candles lit, soft music playing, and we would open the doors to their balcony to let in the salty air that Babette loved so much. It would be *the* most peaceful death I had ever attended. Even as I looked down at the chaos in front of me, it felt unreal that *this* is how things were happening.

About thirty minutes after we arrived, Amanda and Steve walked in. I let out a sigh of relief and watched as Amanda took in the scene of Babette on a stretcher in the hallway, struggling to breathe, as hundreds of people passed by. Amanda took a quick breath before turning on her heel to go find the charge nurse.

"What is wrong with y'all? You have her dying in the hallway? Where is your humanity?" I heard Amanda whisper-yell. I was so grateful to her in that moment. Her admonition worked. A few minutes later, we were ushered into room six, where we were able to relax a bit. Chris brushed Babette's hair back as she breathed heavily, and Tom stood close at her side.

Inelegant as the moment was, CJ and Nick had both been able to say their goodbyes to their mom—but there was still one child we couldn't get ahold of: Chris's brother Eric, the baby of the family, who was in the military. Tom called and called, but he couldn't get through. Finally, he gave up and the three of us sat at Babette's bedside, telling her how much we loved her, waiting for the end.

Finally, as if by some sort of miracle, the phone rang. It was Eric. Tom answered and quickly explained what was happening before placing Eric on speakerphone. "Mom, I love you," I heard him say loud and strong, just as Babette took her final breath.

There was a long moment of silence and then Tom announced through his tears, "Your mom's not here anymore, Eric, but she heard you and she loves you."

Deep sorrow set in as I looked at Babette's now-lifeless body lying small and fragile in this sterile environment. Not only was my mother-in-law gone, but I had failed her.

Albert

DESPITE ALL THE PEOPLE I'D HELPED PASS, BABETTE'S death made me realize that I knew very little about the next steps. My experience ended once a person was handed over to the funeral home. Even though I'd grown up around funerals, it turned out that I was oblivious to all of the decisions entailed in putting them together. Tom didn't want to make all of those decisions by himself, so Chris and I were by his side, helping out however we could as the arrangements were made.

Thankfully, the funeral home walked us through the process, but there were many more choices to make than I had anticipated. What picture did we want for the booklet that is passed out during the service? What Bible passages would Babette want read? What should her obituary say? Did we want the obituary to be printed in her hometown newspaper as well as the local paper? What clothes did she want to be buried in? What kind of flowers should be placed on top of the casket? Where did we want to bury her? What day did we want the funeral to be on? The decisions seemed to go on and on, and the costs crept higher and higher.

One of the more daunting tasks was selecting the casket. The funeral home had them displayed the way I imagine an art museum would display a van Gogh. I held Chris's hand as we stared at them in silence. We only wanted the best for Babette, but the prices of the nicest caskets were more than a little shocking. Neither one of us wanted to suggest how much my father-in-law should spend or insinuate that Babette was worth anything less than the best.

My phone buzzed in my pocket as we were trying to make this impossible decision. "Where are you? I didn't receive a time-off request," the message from Travis read. My mouth hung open. I showed the screen to Chris, who raised his eyebrows in surprise.

"They know exactly where I am! They were the company she passed under! He has her death certificate on his desk!" I hissed, feeling hot tears form behind my eyes.

"Take a deep breath and don't reply right now," Chris advised.

"He expects me to just show up to work after one day off and to start taking care of dying people again? I'm going to quit."

Chris squeezed my hand. "You don't want to quit. You're just hurt. Wait to reply."

I ignored him as I typed a response through my tears. "Sorry, kinda busy looking at caskets right now because, ya know, my mother-in-law died. I have tons of paid time off available. I'll be back in a week. Please don't contact me until then." I pressed send before reading the message back, then showed it to Chris who, to my surprise, snorted in amusement.

"He deserved that. I just didn't want you to regret anything. My mom would be proud of you for standing up for yourself."

I smiled at my husband and rested my head on his arm. "Family is all that matters right now. She taught me that too. Now, let's get back to helping your dad. Want to suggest one in the middle price range?"

Chris nodded as we turned our attention back to funeral planning.

ON MY FIRST DAY back at work a week later, I started wading through emails in my car outside the office. I wasn't ready to face anyone yet. I was still angry at Travis, and I was also feeling anxious about what awaited me inside after the text I'd sent.

I read an email from Steve, which felt like the safest place to start. "Hadley, welcome back," it read. "The funeral was beautiful, a wonderful tribute to a wonderful woman. I wanted you to start your day with this quote: 'What we once deeply loved we can never lose, for all that we love deeply becomes a part of us.' I know you will do amazing things going forward. She is always beside you and will always be there for guidance." I sighed and worried Steve was overestimating me. Right now, I had no desire to do anything, and I still felt like a failure for how Babette's death had occurred. Was I *really* the right person to be providing end-of-life care?

I continued scrolling until I saw another email from our

social worker, Mindy: "We have a young mom with cancer who wants to take some pictures with her kids before she passes. Does anyone have any connections to wig shops? She wants to look as much like her former self as possible." I sighed heavily and looked up to the sky. *That's the first thing you want me to do, huh, Babette?* I thought. A sunbeam shined through my car. Normally, helping out with tasks like this filled me with joy, but not today.

I texted my father-in-law. "Can one of our patients have Babette's wigs?" I asked. He responded almost instantly. "Of course, much better option than them sitting around our house." I emailed Mindy to let her know that if the patient was blond, I had a lot of quality wigs to donate. Feeling overwhelmed, I closed my email and checked the clock. It was time to go in; the morning meeting had already started.

Everyone turned to see who was late when I entered the conference room. Their faces all softened when they saw me. Everyone's face except Travis's, that is. I made a point of nodding at Steve and Dr. Kumar, who had both come to Babette's funeral. I was surprised when Dr. Kumar showed up, sitting in the back of the chapel after hugging both Chris and me and offering his condolences. He was so busy, and it meant the world to me that he took the time to come.

The meeting came and went in a blur. Before I knew it, everyone was gathering their stuff and I heard Cheryl, our bubbly blond marketer, yelling over the noise. "We need everyone's help getting the turkey list complete, so make sure you are asking all of your patients! I need the final lists by the end of next week." Every year, we provided Thanksgiving turkeys to our patients who couldn't afford them on their own so that they could celebrate the holiday.

"Nurses! Wait!" Travis yelled. I paused and put my stuff back down. "We have a new admission. It's a . . . unique situation we don't encounter often. I need to figure out who has the time for it. I know we're all overloaded and stressed, but someone has to take on one more. How many?" he said, pointing at me with his ballpoint pen.

"I have fifteen patients right now, but I don't want anyone with brain cancer. I can't handle it," I said. Without commenting, Travis wrote down fifteen next to my name before continuing around the room.

"Sixteen," Amanda said.

"Fifteen," Jenna said.

"Jenna, Hadley, you're adults and I trust you can make the decision between yourselves. This patient doesn't have brain cancer," Travis said.

"I think the easiest way to decide is to see who already has patients close to this patient's house so there's less travel time," Jenna suggested, looking at me for approval. I nodded in agreement. Travis scratched his head with his index finger before using his whole palm to wipe down his face.

"So, that's the unique part. He is homeless. He lives under the East Creek Bridge." This was certainly a unique situation. I normally wouldn't be the first to volunteer, but I could hear Babette in the back of my mind saying, *Take him. It's the right thing to do.*

"I'll take him," I volunteered.

"Great!" Travis said, clearly surprised at how easy that was.

He handed me the stack of paperwork before exiting the office with Jenna and Amanda. I scanned the doctor's note from the hospital. "Albert, age seventy-seven, kidney failure and diabetes, unknown date of origin, poor historian," I mumbled to myself as I read. "Refused right above-the-knee amputation. Refuses rehabilitation placement. Discharge to hospice." I flipped to the back of the packet to look at his insurance information. It was blank. *Odd*, I thought. *He should at least have Medicare if he is seventy-seven and* definitely *Medicaid if he's homeless.* I picked the packet up and walked over to the social worker's office.

"Hey Mindy, have you seen this new admit packet yet? Mr. Albert?" I asked her. She swiveled around while finishing off the breakfast bar she held in her hand.

"Uh-huh," she said, "I'm working on that Medicaid app now. We'll get him out from under the bridge and into a nursing home. I wish the hospital would have tried a little harder."

I sighed with relief. "Thank you so much."

AS I DROVE, I felt my cheeks flush thinking back to what filling out my own Medicaid application had been like. At my first ob-gyn appointment, I was greeted by a smiling receptionist who asked me for my insurance card. I pulled it out, handed it over, and she gave me a stack of paperwork to fill out in return. A few minutes later, she called me back up to the desk.

"Do you have a different insurance card?"

I felt my stomach churn. "No, does it not work?" I asked.

"I called, and it was canceled," she said.

My insurance plan had been under my dad's name, and he wasn't pleased about my pregnancy. "I'll just cancel the appointment, then. I'll be okay. I feel okay."

The receptionist's eyes shifted to her co-worker. "You need prenatal care. If you don't get it, there's a chance your baby will be taken from you when they're born, due to neglect."

I felt like I was going to have a panic attack. "Okay, I'll get a job and pay out-of-pocket then."

"It's about thirty-five thousand dollars and we need some of it up front."

I had less than a hundred dollars in my bank account and my mom was barely able to make mortgage payments in the wake of her still-recent divorce. There was no way I could ask her.

"I'll sign up for insurance myself," I said.

"You have a preexisting condition now. Your only option is Medicaid."

"What's Medicaid?"

"It's for the poor. It's free."

"Can I have some time?" I asked.

I left the office and sat in my car. I had always been told that state programs were for lazy people, people who wanted to "sit at home and let everyone else work for them." I did not want people to think of me that way, but I also didn't know what other options I had at this point. That night, I filled out the Medicaid application with tears in my eyes. I was determined to get out of this situation and to make life better for me and my child.

I opened a new tab on my computer and started researching different career paths. I even took a quiz titled, "What

Should I Be?" After answering a bunch of personality-based questions, my result popped up on the screen: nursing. I did some more research and then, with a newfound sense of determination and hope, made an appointment with an advisor at the local college. I began to feel better. I had a plan.

A few days later, I was sitting in the community college advisor's office, where I had been waiting for more than an hour. My pregnancy had just started to show and I couldn't afford maternity clothes, so I kept pulling down my shirt as I shifted in the uncomfortable plastic lobby chair. When I was finally called to the advisor's office, she peered at my belly from over her glasses. Looking away, she sifted through the paperwork I had brought with me, including my college transcripts from my freshman year, and then finally put them down and folded her hands in front of her. "Nursing school is very hard to get into," she said.

I nodded. I had already seen the statistics online.

"From what I'm seeing," she continued, "you would need all A's in your prerequisite classes to get in, and it looks like you might have other priorities at the moment."

I nodded again, then said, "I can do this. Please enroll me in the classes."

She sighed heavily as her fingers hovered over her keyboard before placing them back down on the desk again. "How about something easier? Your chances are just so low."

I felt a fire in my belly that I hadn't felt in some time. "I will be a nurse. Enroll me."

She shook her head from side to side in a *tsk-tsk* motion while entering the courses into her computer. When she finished, the advisor handed me my class schedule and said, "I'll be here if you need to drop or change any classes."

I took the paper from her and exited the office, more determined than ever. I was going to prove her wrong.

A few days later, I showed up to the rescheduled ob-gyn appointment, Medicaid card in hand. A different receptionist asked for my insurance card. As I handed over the gold card and stood there waiting for further instructions, I saw her roll her eyes. With her back to me, she told her co-worker, "People who can't afford to be parents shouldn't be allowed to be parents."

My whole body froze. I wanted to run away, but as she turned back around and smiled at me, I couldn't do anything except smile back. I left the office that day knowing that if I ever became a nurse I would never treat someone the way she treated me.

NOW, YEARS LATER, DESPITE the skeptical college advisor and the nasty receptionist, here I was, a successful nurse, and here was an opportunity to keep that promise I had made to myself in the doctor's waiting room.

As I approached the East Creek Bridge, I realized I didn't know how to get below it. On one side of the bridge was a shopping center and on the other was a military-owned beach. Seeing no other option, I made a turn onto the compacted sand and parked next to one of the prominently displayed NO TRESPASSING signs. I gathered my nursing bag and tablet, got out of my car, and hit the lock button at least three times. Still not seeing anyone, I began walking toward the bridge. As I got closer, I saw tents and trash strewn about. I held my hand up to shield my eyes from the sun as my sneakers sunk into the sand with each step.

As I came upon the first tent, I saw a woman crouched down with a stick in her hand, drawing circles in the sand. Her hair was matted and dirty and her T-shirt was worn and flimsy. It was getting cold at night now, and I hoped she had something warm in her tent. As I walked closer, she turned her head to face me.

"Hi there! I'm looking for Albert?"

The woman's scowl turned into a big, toothless grin—and then she began yelling at me. Although she wasn't speaking a different language, her words were incomprehensible. As she yelled and waved the stick around, I instinctively took a step back, scared. I touched my phone in the side pocket of my pants and considered calling Steve to see if he could accompany me.

Just then a shirtless man wearing dirty blue jeans yelled at me from about fifty yards away. "Hey! Are you here for Al?"

I nodded before realizing he probably couldn't see me well. "Yes, I think so. Albert," I yelled back.

As the shirtless man jogged toward me, I felt fearful again, unsure what to expect. He must have read the fear on my face because he said, "Al is right over here. She's harmless, she just can't talk good. I'll show you where he is." The man motioned toward the bridge as he began walking back that way.

I followed him, taking in my surroundings. There were lots of people, sleeping bags, extinguished fires, and bottles strewn over the sand. The shirtless man acknowledged everyone we passed with a nod or wave. During one wave, I noticed multiple scars up and down his arm. His hair was brown, wavy, and unkempt. He was probably in his thirties, and his tanned skin betrayed his living situation, unprotected from the elements. As he walked, he turned back toward me to make sure I was keeping up.

"I'm Gil, by the way."

"Hadley," I replied.

When we arrived at Albert's tent, I noticed a homemade cardboard sign propped up with the words SPREAD LOVE NOT HATE scrawled across it in Sharpie. The tent's flap was open and I could see a man lying on the ground inside. He wasn't wearing shoes and one foot was swollen, the other wrapped in a dirty bandage. The bandage was from the hospital and the date read 10/25, which meant the dressing had not been changed in four days. I knew from Albert's records that his unmanaged diabetes meant that his foot couldn't heal and had become infected. With the right care, this situation would have been preventable.

"Hi! I'm your nurse," I said.

Like Gil, Albert's skin was dark from the sun and his face was heavily lined. Although those lines looked like laugh lines, Albert certainly wasn't laughing right now. He snapped his head up and frowned at me. "What for? I don't need no damn nurse."

I was taken aback. Clearly the hospital told him I was coming, right?

"Well, since you didn't want to do any treatments, they sent me to make sure you're comfortable."

Albert rolled his eyes and put his head back down, not saying anything.

"Man, just try it. I don't want to see you like this. You're hurtin', man," Gil encouraged him. Albert groaned and sat up, scooching out of the tent and putting more pressure on his bandaged appendage than I would have liked in the process. Taking that as a yes, I moved out of the way and pulled the admission paperwork from my nursing bag.

"This will only take a second. I just need a few signatures," I said, fumbling for a pen before realizing I had nothing to write on. Usually I sat at a dining room table with families as we signed the paperwork. I looked around while Albert sat with his head down, looking uncomfortable. Thankfully, Gil understood my predicament and picked up the cardboard sign, handing it to me to use as a writing surface.

As I went through the paperwork, Albert listened and mumbled that he understood what he was consenting to, then signed each piece of paper. When I got to the portion asking about his pain level, he finally looked up. "What would you say your pain level is right now on a scale of one to ten, ten being the worst?" I asked, pen poised and ready to write down his answer.

Albert chuckled, looking at the water, then he looked directly at me. "Ten. But why don't you write down six because every time I say ten you people think I'm looking for drugs."

I paused, unsure what to write. Deciding to leave the box blank for now, I asked Albert if I could order him medications for his pain. He shrugged in response. Reading over the next question, I felt my phone buzz in my pocket. I read a text from Mindy: "I need a copy of his driver's license and bank statements for the Medicaid application." Putting my phone back in my pocket, I said, "That was our social worker. She is working on an application for you so we can get you placed somewhere. Can I send her a picture of your driver's license and bank statements?"

Albert laughed an actual laugh, then said, "Gil, did you hear that?" Turning back to me, he said, "Honey, I don't have a driver's license or a bank account. I don't have a penny to my name."

"Oh, well, I'm sure they will understand. Let me just tell her," I replied, typing Albert's response back to Mindy. A moment later, she wrote back, "It's going to take awhile, then. The computer system won't let me submit without those two documents being uploaded. I'll have to mail it in." I huffed in frustration.

"I'm not going to that nursing home, so you don't have to sweat it," Albert told me. "Finish your questions."

"You have to! You can't stay here!" I protested.

"Why not?"

"It's . . . it's not safe," I whispered.

"What makes you think that being around doctors and nurses makes me feel safe?"

I paused. I was used to people trusting me without question, but I understood where Albert was coming from. I remembered feeling the same way in that ob-gyn's office.

"I shouldn't have assumed. I'm sorry," I said, looking down at his bandaged foot. "Can I change that?" I asked, motioning toward the wound. He nodded. Gil hovered over us, watching my moves in a protective fashion. As I took out my supplies and placed them on a clean cloth, I considered what to say next. It was important to maintain professionalism, but my instincts were telling me that I would need to be a little vulnerable to gain Albert's trust. I put my blue gloves on and began removing the tattered tape from the gauze. "I had a baby at twenty," I told him as I worked. "I wasn't married. I know it's not as serious as your situation, but a lot of people who I trusted shunned me."

"You got a pretty big rock on your finger," he observed, clearly skeptical of my story.

I nodded, now unwrapping the gauze. "I just got married this year. For a long time, I thought no one would love me, like I was damaged goods, but I found a man who does, and he loves my son too."

"Damaged goods? Huh. Yeah, I get that," Albert said, nodding thoughtfully. He paused for a moment as I wrapped his foot, then said, "I would say that maybe we will get along, after all, but I don't know if I can trust anyone stupid enough to wear that huge rock down to a homeless camp." I looked up to see Albert smiling a big smile, clearly joking with me now.

I smiled back just as big and joked, "Hey, now! I did lock my car. That's more than I usually do."

"Stupid white women," he said, shaking his head and chuckling. "I respect you for coming by yourself. No one will mess with you here, and I mean that. They won't harm someone trying to help me. Also, they know that Gil isn't afraid to put them in their place if they get a wild hair." I believed that, especially that Gil would be willing to harm someone with good reason. After I finished dressing Al's wound, I remembered the turkey list.

"Oh yeah! We're giving out cooked turkeys. Can we bring you one in a few weeks?"

"Nah, it's nearing Thanksgiving so there will be loads of people trying to give us food. It's about the only time of year we can count on a hot meal. They'll all be gone in a few weeks, though, so maybe ask again then?"

I nodded, feeling guilty that we didn't offer food other weeks of the year. Before leaving, I handed over the bright orange sheet with the number for our nurse's line. "Use this number like you would use 911. Call us instead. We have a nurse on call 24/7." Then it hit me. This was probably the fifth time I had caught myself having to correct my usual spiel to fit Albert's needs. "Do you have a phone?" I asked. I realized how often I was on autopilot and vowed to make a conscious effort not to be.

"Nah, but there's a pay phone right up the road," Gil said, arms crossed. "I'll make sure it's taken care of."

"Okay, one last thing. I'm guessing our doctor will order medications. I can bring a little safe to keep them in, but are you able to pick them up from a pharmacy?" I asked.

"The CVS is only a mile away. I'll do it," Gil volunteered, placing his hand on Albert's shoulder in reassurance.

"You're a good friend," I said to him, collecting my things.

"We're not friends, we're family here, and we take care of each other."

"I like that. I'll be back in two days, okay?"

They both nodded in assent.

I made the trek back to my car and called Dr. Kumar to get his approval for the medications. He expressed concern about having narcotic medications in that environment, so he suggested ordering a smaller amount than usual. I told him that Gil had to walk two miles round-trip to get the medications.

Dr. Kumar sighed in frustration. "And he won't go to a nursing home?"

"He won't go. His family is with him at the bridge and he wants to be with them when he dies, just like our other patients do," I said, holding firm.

"Okay, I'll order them. Can you count them during the visits, though?"

"Of course," I agreed. "I do that for all of my patients. Thank you."

As I finished up the paperwork and hit submit, I saw an incoming call from the nursing aide, Deja. "Hey! Are you back from your family leave?" she asked as soon as I answered. "Because I think you are, but if not I am *so, so* sorry for calling."

"I'm back. Do you have the new patient, Mr. Albert? I just met him. He's nice."

"Yes. I can go on the visit with you in a couple days if you want?"

"Sounds great! How's the baby?" I asked.

"He's seeing a physical therapist now after the surgery for his scoliosis. It's been really stressful trying to get him to all the appointments between seeing patients."

"I can only imagine. I'm always here if you need me."

As we hung up the phone, I checked the time. I still had about an hour before my next patient. I was near my father-in-law's house, so I ran by to grab the wigs. It was also his first day back at work, so the house was quiet as I rifled through his and Babette's bedroom. His bedroom? I wasn't sure what to call it now. The wigs were displayed on stands, but I chose to put them in a grocery bag instead because something about walking around with Styrofoam heads and real human hair seemed odd.

As I drove to drop off the wigs, I realized that the patient lived on the same street that Reggie had lived on. I wondered who his home had gone to, and hoped that it hadn't gone to one of the many developers in the area. Driving up the street, I noticed a large bulldozer and felt uneasy. I stopped my car in the street, not caring what the workers thought of me, and stared at the cleared land. Reggie's home was completely gone, and so was his neighbor's. Not only that, but they had taken out all of the trees—the same trees that had swayed in the wind as I'd had that last conversation with Lisa. Based on the foundation poured over both pieces of property, it looked like a million-dollar monstrosity was in the works. Exactly what Reggie didn't want.

I drove a few more blocks to the home of the young mom with cancer. Trying to put a smile on my face to hide my annoyance at the developer, I rang the doorbell, grocery bags full of hair in hand. An older woman answered the door.

"Hi, I'm here to drop these off. Um, they are wigs," I said, awkwardly raising up the grocery bag as I spoke.

"Oh, yes! Come in! They're for my daughter. She's right back here." I wasn't expecting to go in, but I obliged and followed the woman back to the bedroom.

"Honey, the nurse from hospice is here with the wigs," she said, motioning for me to enter. I saw a thin, pale woman lying on the bed, wearing pink pajamas and a fuzzy pink hat to match. She gingerly pulled back the covers and got out of bed. Facing me, her expression was one of sincere gratitude.

"Do you want me to put them over here?" I asked, motioning toward the dresser.

"Actually, I'll try them on. If they don't work, I'd rather you keep them so you can give them to someone else."

I nodded. I didn't feel ready to see someone else in Babette's wigs, but I didn't have another choice. I watched as she pulled each wig out of the bag and raked through the hair with her fingers—something I had watched Babette do many times before. After admiring each one, she chose the bright blond wig with the wispy bangs. She removed her hat and placed it on her head. The straight hair fell to right below her shoulders. Standing behind her, I could see her expression in the mirror. There were tears in her eyes, but her smile was so big that it took up most of her face.

"You look like you again," her mom whispered in awe from the doorway. The younger woman turned around to face us, the blond wig swishing as she spun.

"Thank you. This will give my kids some normalcy," she said to me.

I smiled. "I'm so glad." I was happy for her, but also wished more than anything that I could see my mother-in-law putting on her wig and makeup one last time before a family dinner, and hear her talk about how it looked just like her natural hair.

As I left their home, I took one last look at her mother, the person who would soon be in my shoes, experiencing excruciating grief. *Life can be so cruel,* I thought.

———

WHEN I GOT HOME that night, Brody and Chris were on the couch watching TV, Chris still in his scrubs.

"How was your first day back?" I asked as I put my stuff down.

"It was good. Yours?"

"Well, I got a new patient who is homeless. Something he said really stuck with me," I said as I leaned down to kiss the top of Brody's head.

"What's that?"

"He said that people give him food on Thanksgiving, but after that, they just kind of forget about him. I felt so bad about it."

"Well, if you still have him after Thanksgiving, we can give him food when he needs it."

I smiled, feeling some resolution. "Sounds great. Thanks, babe."

Chris got up and pulled out the watering can from under the sink. After his mom's service, the funeral home asked who wanted all the plants that were sent. There were at least eight large houseplants sent from co-workers, friends, and distant family members. All the adult kids looked at each other, but no one volunteered.

Finally Chris said, "We'll take them." I squeezed his hand to indicate that we needed to talk about it first. I had no idea where we would put that many plants. Once we were alone, he turned to me and said, "We have to take them. We can't let them be thrown away." I nodded. I could tell how important this was to him. Now, every few days, I watched Chris lovingly water all the plants, making sure they were healthy—almost like he was making sure that his mom lived on in some way.

A FEW WEEKS LATER, Thanksgiving had come and gone. By now, I'd had many visits with Albert, who told me, "My friends call me Al, so that's what you should call me too." I learned that he had emigrated here from Mexico with his parents when he was a teenager and worked in construction until he became sick. He never explicitly told me if he was a legal immigrant or not, but I drew my own conclusion when he told me that he'd had no benefits to fall back on when he was unable to continue working. Gil was always by his side, reporting on Al's symptoms and even learning how to change his dressing. They never called the on-call line, no matter how many times I reminded them that it was available. Al always waited for my scheduled visits and never complained when I was running late.

One day when I arrived, Al was in visible pain. I asked how long he'd felt like this and he told me it hadn't been long.

Gil immediately interjected. "He's lying. He's been in pain for two days."

I audibly gasped. "Al! Why didn't you call me?"

"I want you to spend time with your family, Ms. Hadley. I don't matter, I'm used to pain."

As I entered the code to his medication safe and pulled out the morphine that the doctor had ordered for emergencies, I explained to Al, "Here's the thing, though: Once we let the pain get this bad, it's harder to treat. It's like we're playing catch-up. It actually makes my job easier when you call me the second that your pain is worse than usual. Okay?"

He nodded, grimacing through the pain. I drew the morphine into the syringe, the smallest amount, and then said, "This is for your pain. Are you okay with taking it?" Al nodded. "It should start working pretty quickly. I'm sorry this is happening to you. We're going to get this under control, I promise." I looked around for some water. Usually I rinsed out the syringe after using it so it didn't get sticky, but there was no sink available to me here. Instead, I put the syringe back into the box and made a mental note to bring another syringe and an unopened bottle of water next time.

"I think I'm going to be sick," Al suddenly said, holding his stomach.

"Have you eaten recently?" I asked.

"No, we haven't had much available lately," Gil said. "I've been giving him everything I can, but it's just not much. I can go look through some trash cans. Give me a minute."

I thought I was going to cry. "No, I have some peanut butter crackers in my car. I'll be right back." When I returned, I opened the crackers for Al and watched as he began nibbling on them.

"Okay, that helped. I can feel the pain easing off too. Thank you, Hadley." He tried to hand me back the rest of the crackers and I shook my head aggressively, telling him to keep them. Before leaving, I showed Gil how to draw up the morphine and administer it, then watched him demonstrate it back to me.

"Promise to call me?" I asked, pointing at Al and Gil.

"Yes, Ms. Hadley. We'll call," Al said, waving goodbye. I

was happy to see that he looked better than he had when I arrived.

I DROVE TO THE office for the weekly interdisciplinary meeting. When I arrived, I waved to Mindy as I passed her office and practically bumped into Travis as he rounded the corner.

"Hey, how's it going with Mr. Albert?" he asked.

"Today was rough. He was in pain and didn't have any food. I'm going to buy some tonight and drop it off tomorrow, so I may have to skip the morning meeting."

Travis's eyes shifted to the empty office to his right and he cocked his head in that direction, indicating that I should follow him in. He shut the door behind him. Confused, I asked, "What's up?"

"So, we can't actually buy things for our patients. The company has strict rules against it."

"I'm not going to let Al starve when I can afford it," I said, looking Travis directly in the eye. I couldn't fathom how he could be okay with a patient not being able to eat when our goal was comfort care.

"I just want you to be aware because you could risk losing your job if corporate found out. I'm not trying to be the bad guy. I'm just trying to protect you," he said, returning my eye contact.

I wasn't in a financial position to lose my job. I didn't respond to Travis as I opened the door and silently walked back to the office with a heavy heart.

———

LATER THAT NIGHT, I told Chris about Al's situation. He immediately suggested that we go buy him food.

"Here's the problem. Travis said I could lose my job if I do that."

Chris cursed underneath his breath, trying not to let Brody hear as he played with some toy trucks nearby. He thought for a moment, then said, "Do it anyway. Screw them."

"I can't lose my job. We need my income and the health insurance."

Chris sighed heavily and ran his fingers through his dark hair.

"Maybe this is one of those moments when I need to learn how to separate my work life from home life, like my therapist says. Let's just go out to dinner," I suggested.

"Okay. Brody, let's get on your jacket," Chris agreed, grabbing the car keys and his own jacket. We went to one of our favorite restaurants near the beach and I was able to forget about work for a bit. Until the food came, that is. When the server placed a heaping pile of nachos in front of us, I looked at Chris. "I don't think I can eat," I said.

"Me neither," he replied. We both picked at the appetizer and left without ordering any entrées. Back at home, I tossed and turned all night, thinking about Al going hungry. In the morning, I woke up to an empty bed. Chris's smiling face greeted me as I walked into the kitchen, where he had a fresh pot of coffee brewing. I was dreading going into work.

"I can drop off Brody today," Chris offered. That was something I usually did, but I appreciated Chris filling in this morning so I could take some extra time to start my day. After showering, dressing, and reviewing my work emails from the night before, I got into my car and placed my purse onto the passenger seat as I always did. I heard a crinkling noise and when I looked over I realized that there were packs of Gold-fish, crackers, and fruit cups in the passenger seat. I smiled and pulled out my phone to text Chris: "Just got in my car. Does this mean what I think it means?"

"Yes. Don't compromise your morals. We will figure it out if you lose your job."

I glanced at the clock on my dashboard. I had planned on going to the morning meeting. If I didn't, it would raise red flags; but if I went, there's no way I'd have time to squeeze a visit with Al in with all of my other patients for the day. Try-ing to figure out a solution, I pulled up the nursing assistants' schedules. Deja had Albert scheduled for today. She usually got her day started early, so there was a chance she was with him now. Nervous, I rang her number. She picked up quickly with a cheerful "Good morning!"

"Is there any chance you're with Mr. Al?" I asked.

"Yup, just got here."

"Do you need any help?" I tried.

"Oh, no ma'am, I can handle it," she replied politely.

"Deja, I need for you to need help today," I said in what I hoped was a convincing tone. "He isn't able to walk anymore and he's a pretty big guy. It might be difficult for you to bathe him without assistance."

There was silence on the other end of the line. For a mo-ment, I thought that maybe Deja had hung up on me. Finally, I heard her say, "You know, my back is hurting this morning. I could email Travis and let him know that I need some help."

I celebrated silently, telling her calmly that I'd be happy to come do that. "Maybe suggest to him that we can do a dual visit and meet that requirement for the week," I told her.

"Got it," she said. Feeling satisfied, but nervous that Travis would see through our ruse, I started driving in the direction of Mr. Al. About ten minutes into my drive, I saw my phone light up with an incoming call from the office.

"Hello?" I answered.

"Hey." It was Travis. "Deja needs some help. Would it be out of your way to go assist her with Mr. Albert quickly?"

I paused, pretending to consider the question for a moment. "I think I can do that," I said, then ended the conversation quickly so I wouldn't give myself away. Buzzing with nervous energy, I drove to the bridge, parked my car, and piled all the food high, using my chin to balance it. I could see Deja waving at me in the distance. As I approached, I placed the food near Al's tent, then looked around for Gil.

"He leaves so Al can have privacy while I'm here bathing him," Deja said, reading my mind.

"Gotcha. Hey, Mr. Al!" I called. He waved, and I noticed he looked worse than he had the day before.

"I brought you some food. Sorry, it's mostly what my son likes, but I can make a grocery store run tonight. Do you want some crackers?" I asked. Mr. Al nodded again without speaking. I tore open a package of crackers and handed them to him one by one. With each cracker he ate, he looked a little better. He washed down every few bites with some bottled water.

"Um, you can't tell anyone I did this," I said to Deja quietly.

Deja laughed. "Where do you think he gets the bottled water from?" she asked with a wink. I looked at her, wide-eyed. "Our secret," she said.

After letting Al finish a few packs of crackers, Deja and I cleaned him up together. Before changing his dressing, I reached into the safe to give Al his pain medication. Changing the dressing always hurt him. I checked to make sure he wasn't running low on medication, but the bottle was still more than half full.

As I was drawing it up, Al stopped me. "No, I don't need it. I don't feel most of my leg anymore," he said. That wasn't a good sign; his condition was worsening. And, sure enough, when I peeled off his old dressing, Al didn't grimace or shift in pain like usual. In fact, it was like he didn't know I was doing it at all.

While I cleaned the wound, Deja observed and handed me supplies as I needed them. "Are you going to do this one day?" Al asked Deja.

"I hope so. Getting there is the tough part," she replied.

"She's going to be an amazing nurse one day," I chimed in. "Only a few more months of being with our company until they will start paying for your schooling, right?" I asked her.

Deja smiled slightly and touched my shoulder without replying. I was confused. Just a few weeks ago, Deja had told me how excited she was to start nursing school and make a better life for her son. Finishing up the dressing, I smiled and asked Mr. Al what else we could do for him.

"Nothing. You two are angels on Earth," he said. Deja and I said our goodbyes and I reminded him to phone the on-call line when he needed us.

As Deja and I began walking back to our cars, I shoved my hands into my jacket pockets to protect them from the cold wind coming off the water. After walking for a minute, Deja broke the silence.

"I'm quitting."

I was shocked. She was the best nursing assistant I had ever worked with. I wanted to respect her decision, but I also wanted to beg her not to go.

"Travis gave me a raise and a promotion to train the other nursing assistants in the area," she continued.

Even more confused, I said, "That's great! You deserve it! You would be *wonderful* at that job."

Deja shook her head. "I can't do it. I've crunched the numbers over and over. The employee health insurance policy for my son and me is nine hundred dollars per month, which means I would make less money than I do right now because our health insurance is free through Medicaid. We already live paycheck to paycheck. If I get a raise, Medicaid says I make too much money and will kick us off. My son is sick. I can't risk us not having health insurance."

I tried to process what she was saying, racking my brain for a solution. "Will they let you stay in your current position and not give you a raise?" I asked.

She shook her head no, her braids brushing against her back. "They already filled it. I took a job with another company. This is my last week."

I sighed heavily. "I'm going to miss you."

"You too, Hadley," Deja replied. "Life is cruel sometimes, huh?"

"It really is."

———

LATER THAT NIGHT, I told Chris about Deja leaving as I did my skin care routine before bed.

"That just sucks. But, hey! At least now you know that if you get fired for the food, you have someone at a different company to vouch for you when you apply for a new job," he joked.

"You're not wrong." I laughed as I splashed water on my face. I put on my pajamas and drifted off to sleep until several hours later when I was suddenly awakened by my ringing phone. I looked at the time: 3:33 A.M. Confused, I squinted at my screen. It was Amanda.

"Hello?" I answered groggily, padding into the bathroom so I wouldn't wake Chris.

"Hadley, I'm so sorry. I know you're not on call, but Mr. Albert's friend called. It sounded really urgent, but when he found out that you weren't on call, he hung up. When I tried to call back, it wouldn't go through."

"Oh my gosh," I gasped.

"I already spoke to Travis and you do not have to go," Amanda said.

I cut her off. "I do. They have never called, even when I've asked them to. I know it's urgent. I'm going." I felt adrenaline pump through my body as I used my phone's flashlight to sift through our drawers for some clean scrubs. Once I was fully dressed, I shook Chris lightly to wake him up.

"Please don't be mad. It's hard to explain, but I have to go see a patient."

"Wha— I thought you weren't on call?"

"I'm not. I have to go, though."

"Your therapist said that this is going to burn you out," he said, more awake now.

"Babe, please trust me. I know something is really wrong. Everyone else has turned their back on this man. I can't do that too."

"Okay, go, I trust you. I just care about you," he said.

"I know. I love you." With that, I quickly kissed him and rushed out the door.

AS I APPROACHED THE bridge, I saw a fire burning and the dark outlines of people huddled around it. I pulled my heavy jacket closer to me against the cold. Despite my surroundings, I wasn't scared. Albert had been right: Everyone knew why I was here, and no one was going to mess with me. As I stepped over the empty bottles and passed people mumbling to themselves, I felt calm. I looked around, trying to make out faces, until I recognized Gil's. I could see his relief as he locked eyes with me. "You came," he said, quickly walking around the firepit toward me.

"Of course I came. What's going on?"

Gil scratched the back of his head. "I'll let him tell you. Please listen to him before you call the doctor."

I nodded, confused, and followed Gil over to Al's tent. Al was lying on the ground, a flimsy blanket draped over him. I set down my nursing bag and got down to Al's level, the sand settling around my body as I sat. "Hey, I'm here," I said softly.

Al opened his eyes and looked at me. "Hadley, I have to tell you something. I know it's a side effect of the medication, but please hear me out first."

I nodded and pulled the sleeves of my jacket down over my cold hands. "I'm all ears. No judgment here."

"I know, but please don't take away my medicine." Al paused, then said, "My momma is here."

I nodded, encouraging him to continue and making sure my face did not react.

"My momma's been dead a long time. I know it's a hallucination, but it's the happiest I've ever been. I'm pain-free and with my momma. Please don't take away the medication."

"Al, what if it's not a hallucination?" I asked.

Al paused and looked past me, into the darkness. After some time, he smiled.

"Do you think it's really my momma? You don't think I'm crazy?" he asked.

"I really do. I don't think you're crazy one bit. Did she tell you anything?"

"She said we're going on a trip and to get lots of rest."

"Well, I think you need to listen to your momma, then," I said with a smile. Gil was nearby, smiling too. *Thank you,* he mouthed to me.

"I'm going to make sure he isn't low on medicine," I told Gil. I reached for the safe and pulled out the morphine. I was shocked. The line was at the exact same spot it had been yesterday morning. Al hadn't taken any pain medication today, yet he was pain-free. There was no way he was experiencing a side effect of medication.

"Well, it's definitely not—" I started to say to Al, then realized he was sleeping soundly.

"I'll let him sleep," I told Gil. "I'll be back in the morning. Well, in a few hours since it's already morning."

"Thank you for treating him like a human," Gil said.

"Thank you for being such an amazing friend. He wouldn't have been able to stay here without your help."

As I walked back up to my car alone, I felt a presence with me, as if a friend was walking alongside me in silence. A comfortable silence that didn't need any words to fill it. I couldn't have felt more safe.

When I got home, I crawled back into bed and tried to sleep for a few more hours. As I lay there, I could feel that same presence with me. It wasn't scary—more like a friend who's in the same room with you, but just out of your line of sight. You know they're there, but you can't see them at the moment.

I groggily hauled myself out of bed a couple of hours later. I could hear Brody playing in the next room. I still had that strange feeling like I wasn't alone. I walked into the kitchen to pour myself some coffee. "I feel like I'm not alone even when I'm alone," I told Chris. "Do you ever feel like that?"

"Oh yeah, not often, but I definitely know what you're talking about."

"Maybe I'm just tired," I said as I walked toward the bedroom to start getting ready for the day. I pulled out clean scrubs from our dresser and put them on, then balled up my pajamas and threw them into the hamper. They landed on top of my dirty scrubs from a few hours ago, and I realized that I hadn't removed my name tag. As I rifled through the hamper, I suddenly felt a gush of wind on the back of my neck. I froze. Too scared to look in the direction of the wind, I waited a moment and then opened up our bedroom door and yelled to Chris, "Hey, does the AC ever just randomly blow air?"

"Uh, yeah, when it kicks on. Why?" he yelled back.

"Oh, never mind. I'm just being silly, then. Thanks." I shut the door again and laughed at myself. I put on my makeup and threw my dirty hair into a bun. After getting Brody dressed, I hoisted him up onto my hip and walked to the car. I felt like I was forgetting something, but I couldn't put my finger on what it was. After dropping him off at school, I suddenly realized that I hadn't taken my name tag off my dirty scrubs. Groaning, I turned back around, knowing I'd be late for the morning meeting, but also knowing that Travis would make me go back home to get it anyway. Dashing inside and ripping the name tag off my scrubs, I glanced at my watch and felt relieved when I realized I'd only be a minute or two late.

As I drove toward the office, the cars in front of me came to a sudden halt. "Ugh!" I groaned aloud in frustration. "Now I'm really going to be late." A few minutes later, the line of cars started to slowly roll forward. After about a mile, I realized what the holdup was: A truck had slammed into the back of another truck. My breath caught in my throat as I looked at the damage, which was severe, but would have been much worse if the car that had been hit wasn't so sturdy. *That could have been me and it could have killed me,* I thought. Thankfully, it looked like all parties were out of their cars and walking around. Suddenly, I was grateful to have forgotten my name tag.

The morning meeting came and went with Travis officially announcing Deja's departure. I pouted in her direction.

"We'll have a sign-up for food for her going-away party," Travis was saying when our receptionist poked her head in the door and looked directly at me. "Mr. Albert passed. His friend just called," she said.

I gathered my things and quietly exited the meeting, then drove toward the bridge.

I ARRIVED TO FIND a beautiful sight. All the people I had come to recognize, who lived with Mr. Al, were gathered around him, praying hand in hand. They parted to let me in, smiling at me politely, their faces streaked with tears. As I pulled out my stethoscope to confirm the time of death, I started my two-minute timer and looked around at all the people who loved Mr. Al. I listened to them quietly pray over him, some with their eyes open and some closed, and I felt so happy that Al got to stay with the people who were like family to him. After two minutes had passed, I noted the time of death and looked up to see Gil a few feet away, sitting on the sand and staring out at the water.

"Hey," I said quietly as I walked up to him.

"Well, we knew this day would come, huh?" he said, choking back tears. "Al was very fond of you. Thanks for caring for him."

"I was very fond of him too," I said, taking a seat next to Gil. "I called a funeral home that will do cremations pro bono. As long as no next of kin come forward, do you want the remains?" I asked.

"Yeah, he wants me to scatter him out here with everyone. You can come too," he said.

"I definitely will."

ONCE THE FUNERAL HOME workers arrived, they carefully placed Al onto their gurney with Gil's assistance. Gil said his final goodbye to his friend with tears running down his face.

"Make sure you let me know when the service is. I will be there. Okay?" I said to Gil.

"I promise."

"So, this isn't goodbye, it's see you later, okay?"

"See you later," Gil said with a half smile.

I waved and walked off. Before I got too far, I heard Gil call out to me, "Oh, Al kept saying the other day that he had a bad feeling about you getting into a car wreck. Make sure you drive safe, okay?"

I froze in my tracks for a few seconds, then turned back around to face Gil. "Thank you," I said. "I will."

Over the years, I've become comfortable with believing and recognizing when things happen, even when I don't know why or have no logical explanation. Looking back, I believe that the presence I felt so strongly that night and the next morning was somehow connected with Al—and that presence was going to make sure I was okay.

Frank

ENTERED THE CONFERENCE ROOM, MAC AND CHEESE in hand, and took in my surroundings. A banner reading WE WILL MISS YOU! hung over the long wooden table. Deja's going-away party was scheduled for during our weekly meeting with Dr. Kumar.

I pulled my pen out of my scrub pocket to sign her card. As I finished writing about how wonderful a nursing aide she was and that no one would ever replace her, Dr. Kumar walked in with his dish.

"That smells amazing!" I said as he placed his plate down next to mine. "What is it?"

"Samosa," he replied. "But you know I can't take credit. My wife made them."

"Well, thank goodness for that," I joked.

Dr. Kumar placed his laptop down, plugging it into the wall behind him. He still had on his white coat from the hospital. As he took it off, he seemed to remember what he wanted to talk to me about. "Oh, I'm helping to start a new program at the hospital," he said.

"Oh yeah?" I replied, looking at my phone, distracted by the emails that seemed to have flooded my inbox within the last half hour.

"Yeah, I think you'll be a good fit for it too. You're coming up on your two-year anniversary in hospice, right?"

"Just passed it a few weeks ago," I told him.

"Well, I want you and Amanda to start doing hospice consultations in the hospital. I've noticed that when our hospital social worker explains hospice, they aren't able to answer most of the family's questions."

"Yeah, that makes sense," I said, nodding.

Travis walked in at the tail end of our conversation and chimed in once Dr. Kumar was done explaining it. "We actually already have a patient for you," Travis said.

"That was quick!"

"Do you want to head there after the meeting?"

"Yeah, I can answer some questions. Easy-peasy," I agreed flippantly.

I TOOK IN THE familiar sights and sounds as I walked into the hospital for the first time since my mother-in-law had passed. The floor looked freshly waxed and the smell of cleaning chemicals was strong, as always. A receptionist sat behind the oval desk, ready to give out directions. I navigated around her, toward the elevators. No one ever questioned where I was going when I was wearing scrubs.

I reviewed what I knew about the patient, Mr. Frank, so

that his family wouldn't have to re-explain everything to me. I had learned firsthand when I was caring for Babette how exhausting and frustrating that could be.

I made my way to room 328, which was spacious and contained a large window and couch. The hospital bed was tilted up at an angle, almost like a chair. A man with a large bandage wrapped around his neck slept there, snoring slightly. On the couch, a woman who looked to be in her sixties sat knitting, her glasses perched on her nose.

"Hi, I'm Hadley from hospice," I said quietly to the woman.

She looked up from her knitting and turned to face me. "Cheryl," she replied, extending her hand. I shook it and asked if I could sit in one of the chairs. She nodded, and I sat, pulling out my accordion folder that held education pamphlets and a pen.

"Before I begin, do you have any questions?" I asked.

"Are we forced to pray and participate in religious things?"

"Absolutely not. We take care of people from all backgrounds. We have a chaplain if you want to speak with him, but there is no obligation to do so."

"Okay," she replied, sounding relieved, "because I made a few calls to get help, but they are all religious organizations that wanted to come and pray for us, and we just aren't comfortable with that."

"What all do you need help with?" I asked. "Because we have a social worker who is great."

"Well, Frank was told this morning that he needs another blood transfusion." I nodded, encouraging her to continue. "It isn't necessary, though, since he is going into hospice. All it will do is buy him a few more days. We don't have insurance, so we would have to pay for it out of pocket. I asked about the cost and have been waiting for an answer, but I'm assuming it's in the thousands."

As she spoke, I mentally went through their options. He was just under the age of sixty-five, which meant he didn't qualify for Medicare yet.

"Did you try Medicaid?" I asked.

"We were denied. We own a vacation rental management company, so money is great in the summer and bad in the winter. Our taxes showed that we made pretty good income last year, fifty thousand dollars, but that went pretty quickly once Frank got sick. I looked into private insurance, but I don't even have the monthly payment they want."

"Well, the good news about hospice is that we take charity patients, so you won't get a bill from us. But I don't think a blood transfusion would be included . . ." I said, trailing off. My thought process was interrupted by Frank, who had started violently coughing. As he did, he grabbed the bandage on his neck. His wife quickly got up and ran over, pressing the bandage down. He stopped and relaxed back into the bed, looking at me.

"Are you from billing?" he asked.

"No, I'm from hospice, just here to answer questions."

"Where the hell is billing?" he asked, clearly annoyed. I didn't blame him. Waiting for someone to tell you if you can afford to live a few more days sounded like torture.

"Let me see what I can do," I said. I walked back into the hallway and found the unit secretary. After explaining to her who I was looking for, she hiked her thumb behind her to a table of scrub-clad women who were typing away on computers.

"Hi," I said as I approached the group of women. "I'm not trying to rush y'all, but does anyone have a status update on the blood transfusion cost for Frank in 328?"

A woman with dark hair twisted neatly on top of her head rifled through some papers before responding. "Yeah, I haven't had a chance to go in yet. They can't afford it. Go ahead and have hospice admit."

"Oh, I'm actually from hospice," I said.

"Great!" she said, placing a large check mark on the paper in front of her. "You tell him, and that's one less thing for me to do." With that, she turned away from me and back to her computer.

"I don't think that's my place," I replied, but she either didn't hear me or she chose not to, because she just continued typing. *Wonderful,* I thought as I walked back into room 328.

"I FOUND A CASE manager who told me that the blood transfusion was, um, out of budget," I informed Frank and Cheryl. "I didn't get an exact number, though."

They looked at each other.

"We could dig into our retirement," Cheryl said.

Frank sighed. "I don't want you to be without money once I'm gone."

"I don't want to lose you, though," she said.

"What's the point of a few more days?" Frank asked. "The outcome's the same. Just sign the lady's paperwork."

Cheryl turned toward me with tears in her eyes.

"I guess that's that, then. Where do I sign?"

I was taken aback by this interaction. I could not imagine having to make this kind of choice. After taking a minute to gather my thoughts, I let them know that the hospital would have Frank transferred home, and I would meet them there to complete the admission process. Cheryl nodded while Frank stared ahead stoically.

A FEW HOURS LATER, I was walking up their driveway with an admission packet in hand. As I rang the doorbell, I stood on the porch and waited for Cheryl to answer.

"Hi, again. I'm sorry, I don't remember your name," Cheryl said as she let me in.

"It's Hadley, but I understand that you have a lot going on. Don't worry about things like that," I told her.

"It's an awful lot," she said, leading me back to their bedroom, where Frank was sleeping soundly. I tried not to disturb him while I did my assessment. Frank had head and neck cancer. A large tumor protruded from his neck, which is what his bandage was covering. I had spoken to Dr. Kumar on the drive over and he instructed me to change the bandage only when I could see blood. It was likely that it was slowly bleeding out. Dr. Kumar warned me that these deaths were rare, and terrible to witness.

After I did all that I could without disturbing Frank's sleep, I woke him up to ask about his pain. He told me that it was well controlled with his fentanyl patch. As I moved down my admission questions, I got to the section about spiritual concerns. I knew that Cheryl didn't want this to be a factor, but I was still required to ask.

"Frank, what would you say your spiritual beliefs are?" I asked him.

"Atheist," he replied. "Nothing happens once I die."

I recorded his response in my tablet. "Do you have any concerns we need to address?" I asked. I asked everyone this question, and atheists simply answered no.

"I mean, I'm scared of what comes next," Frank said, "but I don't think that's anything you can help with. I don't think anything comes next."

"I think more people feel that way than would care to admit," I told him. "I used to be scared of what comes after death, too, and a lot of my patients have said the same thing."

"*Used to*, huh? What changed?" he asked.

I thought through my answer before speaking, wanting to make sure I didn't answer lightly. Growing up, I had believed in the afterlife without question. Following Taylor's death, and throughout most of my late teenage and young adult years, I had questioned that belief. In those years, things felt black-and-white to me. There either was a religious sort of Heaven, or there was nothing. The way I saw it, there was a solid, specific answer for all of this—for life and death—or there was no answer at all. And now, as a hospice nurse, I had witnessed so many things that I couldn't explain away as pure chance or with any sort of medical reasoning. For every story I had about a patient seeing a deceased loved one, or an inexplicable coincidence like the fire Edith had foreseen or the car wreck Al had intuited, my co-workers had ten more. I couldn't ignore the evidence of something more beyond death. To me, *that* was no longer rational.

When I was a child, I was always looking for explanations about why things are the way they are. How could beautiful, miraculous things happen at the same time as all these bad things? As Theresa put it, *What God would allow all these things to happen?* But working in hospice had challenged that worldview. My therapist had made me more comfortable with what we had come to refer to as the In-Between. "It doesn't have to be one way or the other," she had said. I could accept that bad things happened in this world, while also embracing the spiritual moments I experienced in my work and life, and know that they were both equally real.

I FELT READY TO answer Frank's question. "This changed it," I said, gesturing to his bedroom. "Taking care of people like you. Witnessing patients see their deceased loved ones. Seeing their fear wash away before they pass. Coincidences. I think one or two coincidences are just coincidences, but hundreds? I don't think that's a coincidence anymore."

"Maybe you could write a book one day," Frank said with a small smile.

"Maybe." I smiled back at him.

"One caveat though," he said. "You have to include me in it. I want people to know that not everyone believes in an afterlife."

"Deal," I said, offering my pinky finger. We shook on it. I

could tell Frank's voice was wearing out, and I finished the rest of my assessment quickly so he could rest.

As I left their home, I made sure Cheryl didn't have any further questions. She was grateful for the help, but I could tell she was exhausted. I encouraged her to get some rest and to call us if anything came up.

WHEN I DIALED INTO our daily meeting, I briefed the rest of the team on Mr. Frank and made sure to emphasize that he and his wife didn't want anything religious pushed on them. Everyone told me that they understood and I hung up the phone, ready to head home for the night. I thought long and hard about what would happen if Frank bled out, and how traumatizing that would be for Cheryl to see. I prayed that it wouldn't happen, but accepted that these things were out of my hands. This was a skill I had learned from my therapist and that I felt like I was just starting to master. I'm not sure if my therapist would have agreed, but as I sat on the couch that night and watched a movie with Brody and Chris without checking my phone a million times to make sure I hadn't missed a work call, I felt like I was doing much better.

TWO DAYS LATER, I walked up to Frank's home for a visit. Cheryl looked concerned when she opened the door.

"He's talking to people," she told me.

"Okay, that's totally normal," I assured her. "Let's go look at him together so I can explain things better to you."

When we walked into the bedroom, I noticed that Frank was picking at the bandage on his neck. He looked calm, otherwise.

"Honey, the nurse is here," Cheryl said. Frank looked at me and half smiled. "I told her that you've been confused," she said to him.

"I'm not confused. My sister came to visit and you got scared. My sister is not something to be scared of," he replied calmly and with full assurance.

"Your sister is dead," Cheryl said, her voice rising an octave.

I placed my hand on her arm. "Do you have your admission packet?" I asked her. She nodded, wiping her nose with a tissue as she retrieved it from the dresser. She handed it to me and I flipped through the pamphlets until I found the small blue booklet entitled "Gone from My Sight." It had been added to our hospice packets about a year into my job as a hospice nurse because the phenomenon is so frequent, to the point where it's an expected step of a patient's decline.

Opening it up, I showed Cheryl the page that explained that deceased loved ones visiting patients is normal.

"Why, though?" she asked.

I shrugged. "It's one of those things that just happens. I think we all draw our own conclusions."

"We didn't want religion to be brought into this," she said, the frustration evident in her voice. "I told you that."

"This is actually a medical phenomenon. It happens to people no matter what their spiritual beliefs are."

"I mean, I've always thought those people were confused. Frank is not confused. He's happy. How is he happy?" she asked me.

"I wish I had those answers. I've just come to find some comfort in the unknown. All I know is that Frank and others just like him show us that we don't have to be scared. We'll find out for ourselves one day."

"That makes sense to me. I trust him," she said slowly. "We'll find out one day," she echoed, as she knelt at her husband's bedside and held his hand.

SOON AFTER, FRANK SLIPPED into a coma. I told Cheryl what I tell every family member when they ask about the timeline. "It's usually about seventy-two hours from this point. I've seen just a few minutes and I've seen a week, but we can usually accurately say within seventy-two hours."

Cheryl didn't leave Frank's bedside for two days. On day three, I asked her if we could have our volunteer Will come in so that she could rest.

"Do we have to pay for that?" she asked.

"Nope, he doesn't even charge us. He's just a really kind person. I think you'd like him," I told her. She agreed and I called Will while driving to my next patient's home, asking him to come that night so Cheryl could sleep. He agreed and promised to be there at seven. I told him I was on call that night, so he could call me directly with any needs.

"Are you *actually* on call or are you taking an on-call night for Frank?" Will asked me.

"What are you, my therapist now?" I laughed. "I actually am on call. My therapist has been getting on me about overworking and I've stopped doing that."

"I don't believe you," he said.

"Well, you shouldn't because that was a lie—but I *have* cut back a lot," I laughed.

WILL CALLED ME AROUND 10:00 P.M. I had gotten to eat dinner with Chris and Brody and do Brody's nighttime routine, which I was grateful for.

"His bandage is leaking," Will reported. "Should I wake up Cheryl?"

"No!" I said quickly, knowing what she could potentially witness. "I'll be there soon."

I QUIETLY LET MYSELF into Frank and Cheryl's home and crept back to their bedroom, trying my best to not wake up Cheryl, who was sleeping on the living room couch. The bedroom was dark, aside from the bedside table lamp that illuminated Will's papers. When Will wasn't being a Good Samaritan, he was a teacher, and he often did his grading while patients slept.

When my eyes adjusted to the dim light, I could see that Frank's bandage was soaked and his skin was paler than it had been when I'd seen him earlier. It was clear that he was bleeding out slowly, just as Dr. Kumar had warned. I grabbed my gloves and fresh gauze from my bag, as well as a small trash can from the connected bathroom, which I placed by my feet at Frank's bedside. I removed the old gauze and quickly pressed the new gauze to his neck, only to have the clean dressing soaked through within a few minutes. I had no choice but to stand guard and change out the gauze every few minutes. As I stood there applying pressure to Frank's neck, I noticed that Will was watching me.

"I think it's really great that you do this," I said to him softly. "I don't think I've ever told you how much everyone appreciates you."

He shrugged. "I do it for myself."

"You're humble. There's no way you do this for yourself."

"Want to hear a story?" he asked. I nodded, and Will continued. "My mom passed away when I was a teenager."

"I'm so sorry," I said, but Will held his hand up to stop me.

"I wasn't there," he said. "We hadn't spoken in a year. We got into an argument when I came out to her, and stopped speaking after that. She died alone. This is my way of making things right: not letting anyone else die alone."

I let the weight of his words hit me as I changed out Frank's gauze once again. I wanted to tell Will that it wasn't his fault, but it didn't feel right to share my opinion—he hadn't asked. Instead, I simply told him that it's a wonderful thing that he does, no matter why he does it. He went back to grading papers as I stood there holding Frank's neck.

Lately, I had been practicing coming from a place of empathy rather than sympathy. My therapist and I talked a lot about this too. For so long—even dating back to my earliest days in the ER—I had functioned from a place of sympathy. I put myself in my patient's or their caregiver's shoes; I put myself in the shoes of people like Will. I felt their pain, I felt their loss, and it *affected* me deeply. To be honest, I think this ability to feel what other people are feeling is part of what makes me a good nurse, and especially a good hospice nurse. But it also takes a personal toll, and I'm sure it's one of the reasons why nurses experience so many mental health challenges and don't last for long in the field. In fact, only one out of every four hospice nurses makes it beyond five years, from what I've heard.

Empathy, on the other hand, is the ability to feel for a person and their situation without being personally affected by it. Empathy allows me to be present and compassionate without taking on a situation as my own, and it has allowed me to continue being a good nurse without burning out or engaging in the dark humor that so many people in my profession do, for their own sanity. It has allowed me to be a witness to one of the most important moments in a person and their loved ones' lives.

I *wanted* to keep doing this work. I wanted to continue helping people stay in their homes, getting to know their stories and their families and their pets in the process. I wanted to keep being a part of facilitating a peaceful environment in these important last days, and allowing people in my own life in, while taking care of myself in the process.

FRANK PASSED WITH WILL and me there. When his heart stopped, so did the bleeding. I quickly disposed of the contents of the overflowing trash and went to get Cheryl so she could say goodbye. She only had one question: "Was it peaceful?"

I answered as honestly as I could. "It was one of the most peaceful passings I've ever witnessed."

Adam

I WASN'T HAPPY WHEN I WAS ASSIGNED TO CARE FOR Adam.

"Did you call Travis about this before calling me?" I asked the call center nurse who had just informed me that I would be caring for a patient with brain cancer.

"Yes. He is aware," she replied, sounding confused.

I hung up and immediately dialed Travis's number. "I have told you many times that I'm not caring for brain cancer patients. I made that boundary very clear," I told him as soon as he picked up the phone.

"I know, I know. There's literally no one else that can do it. Please," he said.

I hung up on him, fuming. The thought of caring for people with brain cancer, witnessing the experience Babette should have had, made me feel sick to my stomach. It had been my single most important job, and in the end I couldn't do it. Chris and my therapist had tried to assure me that it

wasn't my fault, but six months later I was still holding on to
the immense guilt I felt about the situation.

AS I PULLED INTO the parking lot of the hospital, I took
deep breaths to try to center myself, but it wasn't working. I
wanted to scream. I walked into the hospital for the second
time since Babette had passed and asked the receptionist what
room my patient was in.

"He's in emergency room six," she directed me.

Of course. The same room my mother-in-law had died in.

As always, the emergency department was busy. Nurses
were running around, babies were crying, and there were so
many different beeping noises that it was impossible to figure
out how the nurses could distinguish one from another. It was
so different from the quiet homes I was now used to.

When I got to room six, I took another deep breath. The
patient in the bed, who I assumed was Adam, couldn't have
been a day over thirty-five. He had on a hospital gown with
tons of wires coming out from underneath it, and appeared to
be either in a coma or sleeping. A woman with straight dirty-
blond hair sat in a plastic chair next to him, holding his hand
and watching the monitors. On the other chair sat a young
boy, probably six or seven, completely immersed in his Game
Boy.

"Hi, I'm Hadley, from hospice," I said, making sure that
my voice sounded even.

"Oh, hi!" the woman greeted me, getting up to shake my
hand. "I'm Jillian."

"I apologize, but I didn't get too much information sent to

me." I turned to the nurse who was charting on a computer set up in the room. "Can you give me a quick rundown?" I asked her.

"Yeah," the nurse replied, snapping her bubble gum. "He got here about an hour ago. Brain cancer. Nothing we can do. That's why you're here."

Surprised by her callousness—especially with this young patient's wife and son in the room—I nodded and told her I could handle it. I sat down in the last open chair in the room and turned toward Jillian. "Can you tell me more? I know it's tough to do."

She gulped and started telling the story. Adam had been working as a real estate agent when he started getting head-aches. He had no other medical issues whatsoever. Then one day, he fainted while showing a house and the client called an ambulance. In the emergency room, they discovered a golf ball–sized tumor. Adam started chemotherapy and things were looking okay for a little while.

"I can't give a specific day when things changed. It was gradual," Jillian said.

I nodded. "I know exactly what you mean."

"He stopped eating much and fell once," she continued, before pausing for a second. "Wait. Most people don't know what I mean when I say that. Have you had a lot of patients with brain cancer?"

I stopped taking notes and looked up. I considered telling her about Babette, but decided against it. "Yes," I said instead.

"That makes me feel so much better," she sighed, touching my arm. I softened a bit. "Anyway, he just got worse and worse until he was like this," she said. "I called 911 and now we're here. No one ever mentioned hospice to us. I have no idea what to do. I'm only twenty-seven," she said.

"Me too," I said, without thinking. I wasn't used to caring for people my age, and her husband and son seemed to be the same ages as Chris and Brody, which made it even weirder.

"Why in the world would you do this job?" she asked me. Then she backtracked, embarrassed by her candor. "I shouldn't have said it like that. I am so appreciative that there are people like you, but I could never."

I shrugged. If I could speak candidly, I would have told Jillian that I couldn't imagine being in *her* shoes—a soon-to-be-widow in her twenties. It pained me to even think about.

"Is it important to you that he passes at home?" I asked her.

"I'd actually prefer for him to be anywhere else," Jillian said, gesturing toward the little boy. "I don't want our son to have those memories."

I understood, but wished there was a better place for people to go than the hospital. Our company had an inpatient unit, which wasn't much better, but it was still probably their best bet.

"We have a place he can go," I offered. "It's similar to here, but it's under our hospice company. Let me just make a quick call."

"Oh, wonderful. Thank you!"

I dialed the inpatient unit, and when the nurse answered I started to explain the situation. She cut me off, saying, "We're full, baby doll."

"Full?" I asked, bewildered. "You're never full!"

"We are now. Last time this happened we kept the patient

at the hospital, but still admitted them to hospice. You can advise the nurses how to care for him."

"Oh, okay, thank you." I hung up and let Jillian know what the plan was. As soon as she was on board, we went through the necessary paperwork. When I pulled out the bright yellow DO NOT RESUSCITATE order, I paused, remembering Babette, then took a deep breath, "I know this seems like a scary piece of paper and it is very serious, but I want you to know that if you decide to sign this, it does not affect any care we will give Adam up until he passes."

She nodded. "I understand. That's what he wants. We talked about this." Jillian stared at the paper, pen in hand, but she didn't move.

"Do you have any questions?" I asked her after a few minutes. She looked at me and I saw that tears were streaming down her cheeks.

"I feel like I'm signing his death certificate, like I'm okay with him dying—but I'm not," she said, placing the pen down and crying harder. I put my arm around her, trying to comfort her while tears welled in my own eyes. She let her body weight rest against me as she cried. After a few minutes, with her head still on my shoulder, she picked up the pen and signed the paper through her tears, apologizing to me. I glanced over at her son, happy to see he was still occupied with his Game Boy.

"Never apologize. The way you're reacting is normal," I reassured her. As she composed herself and sat up straighter, we finished the last few pieces of paperwork.

After asking a few different people which case manager

was assigned to room six, I finally found the right person. I explained to her that our inpatient unit was full, and that Adam probably didn't have much time left.

"We can transfer him up to the third floor so it's not as chaotic," she said.

I exhaled. "That would be wonderful." I went back into room six and noticed that their son was gone.

"His grandparents came to get him. I thought it would be for the best," Jillian said, as if reading my mind. A moment later, a man came in to transport Adam upstairs. Although Adam was over six feet tall, his disease had caused him to lose so much weight that it only took me and one other nurse to transfer him to the bed. He was probably 120 pounds, if not less.

Once we were settled on the third floor, the nurse came in and began placing the blood pressure cuff around Adam's right arm. I assumed that she needed only one reading, but she kept it there as she began putting sticky pads onto his chest to read his heart rhythm.

"Those aren't staying on, right?" I asked the nurse.

"Yeah, of course they are," she replied.

"I'm sure you didn't know, because it just happened, but he's actually on hospice."

"So?" she asked, raising an eyebrow.

"Well, our goal is comfort, so taking the occasional vital sign is fine, but we don't want him to be hooked up to tons of monitors all the time."

The nurse sighed and began taking all the devices off of him. "I don't think they'll allow it," she said, "but we'll see."

She exited the room and Jillian found another chair to pull up to Adam's side.

"Hospice nurse, come here," a curt voice called from the doorway. Confused, I excused myself and made my way into the hall, where I found a medical-surgical unit doctor.

"We keep all patients on a monitor," he said sternly. "I don't care if he's on hospice."

A few years ago, when I was new to this work, I would have backed down without a fight. But now I knew what was right and wrong, and felt confident that I could explain my reasoning.

"If you were dying, would you want to be hooked up to a bunch of monitors?" I asked him.

"I don't do hypothetical situations. Policy is policy," he said, raising his voice. I got the impression that nurses didn't challenge him very often.

"What's going on?" I heard from behind me. Turning around, I saw Dr. Kumar.

"Is this your nurse?" the now-angry doctor asked.

"Yes, what's wrong?"

"Apparently, Little Miss thinks she's above our policy of having patients on monitors," the doctor said, waving his arms in a way that was clearly meant to demean me.

Dr. Kumar looked at me before turning back to the doctor. "What is your reason for having the patient on the monitor?"

"The same exact policy you follow," the doctor responded.

"And what's Hadley's reason for not having it?" he asked.

"Comfort," the doctor replied dismissively.

"All right. Let's say the patient's heart rate drops. Are you going to treat it?"

"No," the doctor responded.

"Are you going to do anything if any of those readings are abnormal?" Dr. Kumar asked.

"No," he replied, looking away as if he was hoping to make an escape.

"Then I don't see a reason for the monitoring. We don't make people uncomfortable for no reason, do we?"

"No," the doctor said one last time, looking down at the floor.

Dr. Kumar squeezed my arm and I went back into Adam's room. I was grateful that he'd been there, but confident that I could have stood up for myself. Still, I was pleased with the outcome. The thought occurred to me that I really was meant to be doing this work.

My good feelings quickly faded as I turned back to Jillian. She had draped herself over her husband's body, trying to get close to him. I touched her back.

"I think it's close," she said, her face wet with tears. I looked down at Adam. There were long pauses between his breaths.

"Do you want to get into bed with him?" I asked her.

"Can I?"

I nodded and brought the rail down for her so she could climb in. Jillian laid her head on his chest and began singing to him. I stood to the side, out of her way, but still there. Her beautiful voice filled the room as she softly sang "Hallelujah," one of Babette's favorites. As Jillian reached the last chorus, Adam took his last breath. It was a beautiful, if heartbreaking, moment that I felt lucky to witness.

———

WHEN I GOT HOME that night, Chris was at the kitchen counter eating a bag of chips. I ran up to him and hugged him harder than I ever had before.

"Rough day, babe?" he asked.

I felt tears gathering behind my eyes. "I had a patient your age. He had a wife and a little boy. He passed. Brain cancer. At the hospital, but he wanted to be there," I rambled. "I just don't ever want to lose you."

"I don't ever want to lose you either, babe," Chris said soothingly, kissing my forehead. "What do you mean he wanted to be there?"

I sighed deeply before answering. "Like, he wanted to pass at the hospital. Unlike your mom, who I was supposed to take care of at home."

"I've been thinking about that," he said. "I think it was meant to happen as it did."

"What do you mean?" I asked.

"Well, if the medicine wasn't forgotten, then you wouldn't have gone to the hospital. If the hurricane didn't happen, you wouldn't have gone to that *specific* hospital, and I would have been working far away. If none of that happened, then she would have been at home."

"Right, that's what was supposed to happen," I said.

"Here's the thing though: I wouldn't have been there. I would have been at another clinic and I would have missed her death. I truly believe that everything happened for a reason."

"Everything happens for a reason," I echoed, realizing, in that moment, that I really believed it.

Conclusion

BECAUSE I WORK SO CLOSELY WITH PEOPLE WHO ARE on the brink of stepping into the great unknown, I'm often asked what I believe in. As you've read, it's been a journey. I have cared for enough end-of-life patients with varying religious backgrounds to believe that how you live your life is more important than what you believe in. I've seen many people live wonderful, fulfilling lives, both with religion and without. I don't think one way is better than the other. What I *do* think is important, though, is finding inner peace and happiness—whatever that means for you. In my experience, the people who are happiest at the end of their life are those who have achieved a sense of peace in regard to how they've lived, and who are comfortable in their belief about what comes next.

I've also learned that, no matter what you believe, everyone dies the same way. I've seen just as many patients who aren't religious and don't believe in an afterlife have end-of-life visitations from loved ones as I have those who do believe in a life

after this one. Having said that, I don't think that we can explain everything that happens here on Earth, much less whatever comes after we physically leave our bodies. I do believe
that our loved ones come to get us when we pass, and I don't
believe that's the result of a chemical reaction in our brain in
those final hours. There's a big difference between hallucinations and the sort of visitations described in this book—I've
seen them both, and they're not the same. While hallucinations can be anything from spiders on the wall to the house
morphing around you, visitations are lucid and matter-of-fact
to the patient who's describing them. While hallucinations
can incite anxiety or fear, visitations bring with them a sense
of calm and peace.

Knowing all of this, I've found my peace and happiness in
the In-Between. I lean on the religious experiences I've had,
such as the one in church when I first discovered I was pregnant. I acknowledge the pain and suffering in the world, such
as what I saw while interning in the ER. And the similarities
among my patients' various end-of-life experiences have led
me to conclude that there is *something* after this life. Knowing
that I am being guided, remembering that we never know
what others around us are going through, and having confidence that this life isn't the end have all helped me live in a
way that I believe I will be proud of when I get to the end of
my own life, whether that be tomorrow or seventy years from
now.

I feel privileged to continue doing this work that I stum-
bled into accidentally, but that I believe is my calling. Today I
work part-time, balancing my work with being a mom to not
just Brody, but also the two daughters Chris and I have wel-

comed since our wedding (the second of whom has been bak-
ing in my belly as I've written this book).

I'm no longer the new nurse—and, in fact, I'm sort of a
veteran at this point, since the tenure of a hospice nurse is
usually brief—but I'm often still the youngest. This work has
profoundly changed not only who I am as a nurse, but as a
person. I didn't go into this specialty expecting to change at
all, yet when I look back, I'm able to see how different I am
now, and how my outlook on life has been profoundly shaped
by my work and my patients.

While I recognize the value and importance of my work
(and that of all hospice and palliative care professionals), our
patients help us just as much as we help them. I've had the
unique opportunity to surround myself with people at the end
of their life. They are usually aware of their impending death
and at a point where they're reflecting on all the experiences
that have, collectively, made a life. Many of these people are
also at a point where they're eager to share their most impact-
ful advice. And that's right when I meet them.

I take their wisdom and the stories they have chosen to
share with me very seriously. I have let them change me. And
that is why I always, *always* eat the cake.

Acknowledgments

THIS BOOK WOULD NOT HAVE BEEN POSSIBLE WITH-out my husband, Chris. From taking over drop-off and pick-up duties and countless bedtime routines to providing me companionship on the couch as I wrote late into the night and a listening ear as I worked through the more difficult memories from my childhood: the quiet but important contributions that you gave on a daily basis did not go unnoticed.

I could never repay my mom for all she did for me in those frightening, uncertain years in my early twenties. When other family members turned their backs, you opened your arms and let me know that you would never leave my side.

Someone only briefly mentioned in this book but so important to me during those difficult nursing school years is my friend Summer. I will never forget our conversation when I thought I might drop out of nursing school. I expected you to support me and whatever decision I made. I was wrong. Instead, you told me no. You told me that dropping out was not an option, that you wouldn't entertain the idea and that we needed to brainstorm ways for me to graduate instead. I do not believe that I would be a nurse today without you.

On that note, I want to thank every nursing professor I had at Northwest Florida State College. While most nurses have horror stories of nursing school professors, I do not. Although you never went easy on any of us, I can confidently say that you prepared me for my first job in nursing not only in clinical skills but in how to properly care for a person as a whole, not just as a patient. It's evident that you also care about making your students into the best nurses possible and that it's not just a job for you.

Thank you to everyone at Verve Talent, specifically Noah. When I met you two years ago, still very new to the media industry, I felt very overwhelmed and intimidated. You and your team have always cared about me as a person first and foremost, and I will always be in your debt. From speaking to other authors, I recently learned that being able to tell your literary agent "I'm so anxious I'm going to throw up" and them calming you down like a therapist is not the norm, but thankfully it is for me (haha). I'm grateful for you for making this whole experience not only bearable but fun.

Thank you to Sara and the entire team at Ballantine. Thank you for taking a chance on a young, new author. Writing down such vulnerable experiences is terrifying, and I appreciate you for always making me feel safe and supported.

And finally to my three sweet children Brody, Callie, and Aristea. I would go to the ends of the earth for you. I hope I made you proud.

A SPECIAL THANK-YOU

I've shared the stories of the twelve patients included in these pages for different reasons, for the different lessons they've taught me. I'm grateful to each and every one of them.

Glenda, as my first hospice death, you laid the foundation for every patient who came after. You were my first introduction to what I now call the In-Between. I appreciate you for so openly sharing your experiences with me, so that I could better understand the differences between hallucinations and seeing deceased loved ones, as you did, and begin my journey to understanding what so many go through at the end of their life.

Carl. Oh, Carl. I could type forever and never come close to what I would share with you if we could be in the same room again today. Thank you for trusting me and allowing me to form a beautiful relationship with you and your wife. Every single day you inspire me to show up as that young, eager nurse determined to make meaningful connections with my patients. I hope you and Anna are dancing together in Heaven. I have two little girls now, and I think of you and your wife often as we move through life. The heartbreak that you two must have endured and continued on with is unimaginable. I miss you, but I understand now more than ever the happiness you must have felt to have Anna welcome you into the after-life.

Thank you, Sue, for openly discussing your beliefs with me and sharing your stories—both the highs and the lows. Those quiet moments watering your plants and folding your laundry

gave me an opportunity to slow down for a moment and re-
flect on my own beliefs. I now understand that no matter
what anyone believes, the happiest people are the ones at
peace with their own beliefs.

Sandra, you and your husband helped me better understand that money, luck, and circumstances do not change how
things end. I now understand that achieving the "picture-
perfect" life, like I believe you two had, will not prevent the
inevitable fact that we all die. What I should have been aspir-
ing to, instead, is the selfless love that you two had for each
other and the people you encountered in life. Thank you for
trusting me to care for you. I hope to follow in your footsteps,
not because of the size of your house, but because of how you
treated people and devoted your life to the service of others.

Elizabeth, I wish you didn't have to go so soon. Your wisdom and positive outlook on life, even in the toughest of situations, has inspired millions. I was stunned at the response I
received when I shared your story on my TikTok account, and
how deeply and vastly it resonated. In fact, I even heard from
a few people who had your words tattooed on them as a constant reminder. Thank you for being so vulnerable with me
and allowing me to form a different outlook than what I had
been taught. Looking back after so many years recovered, I
feel silly for wasting as much time as I did worrying about my
weight instead of "eating the cake."

Edith, you showed me that dementia and Alzheimer's
aren't as black-and-white as I had previously believed. I now
understand that there are factors outside of what we understand that allowed you to defy the rigid boundaries of your
diagnosis. I always remember you while caring for patients

with dementia, and make sure to verbalize what I'm doing and why, just as I would with any other patient, regardless of their diagnosis.

Reggie and Lisa, I have replayed the encounters I had with you so many times, not only with my therapist but also in my own mind. For so long, I felt like it was a puzzle I could piece together: *If only I could go back and figure out the split-second when I went wrong, then I could make sure Lisa's death never happened.* But because of both of you, I have since learned that none of us are as in control as we think we are. Although I wish your story had ended differently, it did finally allow me to seek out the therapy I needed. That therapy has changed how I handle difficulties in all areas of my life, including my marriage, my kids, my work, and my family. Although I wish that Lisa could be alongside me on that journey, I understand that all I can do is look forward. I hope that your story will live on to encourage anyone reading this book who may also need help to seek it without fear of judgment.

Lily, although I only knew you and Allison for a short amount of time, your story has inspired me in so many ways. Not only did I examine my own life and wonder who would be that friend for me, but it has encouraged me to *be that friend.* I've learned that all friendships aren't meant to last a lifetime, and it's okay if some friendships are only for a moment. It's okay to let some friendships fade, without resentment, to make room for those lifelong friends.

My wonderful mother-in-law Babette, father-in-law, sister-in-law, brothers-in-law, and husband welcomed Brody and me into their family with open arms during the most difficult time in their lives. While I feared that no one would accept a single mother, they were all in the process of losing the mom in their family. The love that they all showed during and despite those times will never be lost on me, and I know that so much of that love and acceptance of others was learned from Babette. Babette, I often think of you and hope I make you proud, both as a nurse and as a mom. I know that you continue to watch over Brody, Chris, and me, and I have no doubt that you handpicked the two little girls our family has been blessed with. I will make sure that they know you and your love as they grow.

Albert, you allowed me to examine my morals in a way that I previously had not. Until I met you, I didn't even realize how much I did on autopilot, all the way from the admission process to following upper management's instructions without question. I've since learned how important it is to be a human first and an employee second. Since caring for you, I've changed how I operate as a nurse. I may not be employee of the month anymore, but I don't worry about my morals being compromised—and that matters so much more to me.

Frank, that day when we spoke in your bedroom, I never dreamed that I would actually ever get to write this book. Although I laughed at the ridiculousness of that pinky promise, I'm sure you're the one laughing now. I often wonder if you somehow knew. Your unwavering belief in, well, no beliefs has allowed me to better understand and explain to others that no matter what your beliefs—or lack thereof—your loved ones will still come to get you.

I can never properly explain the array of emotions I felt caring for you, Adam. You were my first glioblastoma patient after losing my mother-in-law, and your family also mirrored mine in appearance. You were a true test of my ability to separate my work life and my personal life. I have since come to understand that our having a personal connection allowed me to be a better nurse and advocate for you, because I had an understanding as a caregiver that others didn't. Because of you, not only do I now always volunteer to take patients with glioblastoma, but I have a better understanding that work life and personal life don't have to be completely separate. As with so many other things, it's okay if there's an in-between.

About the Author

HADLEY VLAHOS, RN, is a hospice registered nurse, mother, and wife whose husband also works in the medical field as a doctor of physical therapy. Vlahos started her career as a registered nurse at twenty-two. As a hospice nurse, she now visits people at their homes while also educating and sharing stories about hospice care on social media, where she has more than a million followers.

TikTok: @nursehadley
Instagram: @nursehadley

About the Type

This book was set in Caslon, a typeface first designed in 1722 by William Caslon (1692–1766). Its widespread use by most English printers in the early eighteenth century soon supplanted the Dutch typefaces that had formerly prevailed. The roman is considered a "workhorse" typeface due to its pleasant, open appearance, while the italic is exceedingly decorative.